Manual of Strabismus Surgery

Commissioning editor: Nick Mowat, Paul Fam
Development editor: Zöe A. Youd
Production Controller: Chris Jarvis
Desk editor: Claire Hutchins
Cover designer: Fred Rose

Manual of Strabismus Surgery

Caroline MacEwen and Richard Gregson

with thanks to Irene Fleming

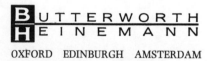

BUTTERWORTH
HEINEMANN

OXFORD   EDINBURGH   AMSTERDAM

BUTTERWORTH-HEINEMANN, an imprint of Elsevier Limited

First published 2003

ISBN 0 7506 5248 9

British Library Cataloguing in Publication Data
A catalogue record for this book is available from the British Library

Library of Congress Cataloging in Publication Data
A catalog record for this book is available from the Library of Congress

Note
Medical knowledge is constantly changing. As new information becomes available, changes in treatment, procedures, equipment and the use of drugs become necessary. The author/contributors and the publishers have taken great care to ensure that the information given in this text is accurate and up to date. However, readers are strongly advised to confirm that the information, especially with regard to drug usage, complies with the latest legislation and standards of practice.

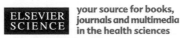

ELSEVIER SCIENCE   your source for books, journals and multimedia in the health sciences
www.elsevierhealth.com

Data manipulation by David Gregson Associates, Beccles, Suffolk
Printed in Great Britain by Martins of Berwick on Tweed

The
Publisher's
policy is to use
**paper manufactured
from sustainable forests**

II

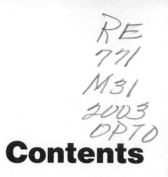

Contents

Foreword

I am honoured and privileged to be asked to provide a foreword for this manual of strabismus surgery. Both authors trained with the Strabismus and Paediatric Service at Moorfields Eye Hospital and have gone on to become distinguished members of the strabismus community in the UK, Europe and internationally.

Many trainees in ophthalmology find the study of strabismus daunting. It may involve the examination of restive children, the reassurance of nervous parents and the awareness that one's orthoptic colleagues know a great deal more than oneself. Other problems include the difficulty encountered in most training programmes of finding out what happened to the patients on whom one has operated, and the real decline in numbers of strabismus operations being performed, which has reduced the opportunity for trainees to learn techniques by performing them under expert supervision. Finally, the terminology may cause some difficulties to the beginner.

Nevertheless, there seems no immediate prospect of patients with ocular motility disorders disappearing from our clinics, and while there is no substitute for practical experience of management, a good book may go a long way towards providing a logical basis for assessment and management of patients. The authors have certainly provided such a text. It is, as they state, a manual of strabismus management, not just of strabismus surgery, and they give clear advice on the management of common and rare types of strabismus.

The book is divided into three logically arranged sections. The first, 'General Principles', outlines assessment of the patient, non-surgical management, principles of surgery and surgical anatomy. While not replacing the fuller discussion available in specialist orthoptics texts, this section makes clear the essential principles of examination, measurement and conservative therapy. The second section 'What to do', identifies specific sub-types of strabismus, their assessment and management. Here the authors describe and classify all types of concomitant, paralytic and restrictive strabismus, in addition to congenital and acquired nystagmus. There are copious and clear management algorithms to aid decision-making in the more complex types of strabismus. The final section, 'How to do it', gives a very clear and copiously illustrated account of all current surgical procedures for management of strabismus, in addition to detailed advice on the applications of botulinum toxin for treatment of ocular motility disorders, and the avoidance and management of the complications of strabismus surgery.

This approach has the great merit of being problem-related, allowing the reader to find the disorder that he or she requires to treat, but naturally also requires a certain amount of cross-referencing within the text to avoid repetition. This is effective and well-organized, and should not cause any difficulty for the reader. The surgical diagrams are clear and thoroughly annotated, so should provide useful guidance for the surgeon attempting an unfamiliar novel procedure.

The bibliography is well chosen for each topic, without attempting to be excessively comprehensive. Readers wishing to expand their knowledge will find following up the references extremely worthwhile.

Finally, although there is not, and never has been, a 'magic formula' for strabismus surgery and its effects, the appendix gives useful and sensible advice on the alignment effect of various procedures on ocular muscles. If read in conjunction with the main text, which gives specific advice on when to aim for deliberate over- or under-correction, the reader is unlikely to get into major difficulties.

No book, however well written, is a substitute for practical experience and our patients are always our best teachers. The authors clearly recognize this, and I hope that some of their future readers will be inspired to follow them into this endlessly fascinating area of ophthalmology, where one can frequently do a great deal to relieve patients' complaints and abolish their troublesome symptoms.

The authors are to be congratulated on their hard work and achievement, and I fully expect their book will have the success that it deserves.

John Lee
Consultant Ophthalmic Surgeon
and Director of Education
Moorfields Eye Hospital

Preface

Despite its title, this book is not all about surgery. Much of the management of strabismus is non-surgical and we hope that we have covered this in the text.

We feel, however, that most books about strabismus have been a little light on the precise ways to perform squint surgery and we hope that we have produced a text that gives a step-by-step guide to this. The aim is to steer the ophthalmologist without a specialist interest in strabismus towards the correct initial surgical treatment, and to give the non-operating specialist (e.g. orthoptist) enough information so that any of the patient's queries could be answered.

To this end the book is divided into three parts:

- **Part 1** provides a background to strabismus. This is not an orthoptic text, but is a practical background introduction to strabismus surgery;
- **Part 2** is an overview of common types of strabismus and provides a step-by-step guide to surgical options and how to decide what to do (and what not to do!);
- **Part 3** describes how to perform the operations. As a number of different conditions require the same surgical procedure and as one condition may have a number of surgical options, depending on clinical findings, there is a great deal of cross referencing between Parts 2 and 3.

The methods advocated in this book are based on the teaching of John Lee and Peter Fells at Moorfields Eye Hospital, under whom both the authors trained in strabismus and ocular motility. These techniques have been further modified over the past decade and have been used as a guide for specialist registrar training in our units. There are many different ways to perform squint surgery, but this is a system that has worked for us for many years.

CM, RG
2003

Acknowledgements

We would like to thank the orthoptic departments of Ninewells Hospital and Queens Medical Centre for advice and encouragment, our specialist registrars who have helped to make the text more understandable, and Lynda Rose for secretarial support. Special thanks to Mr John Lee who read the text and gave us valuable advice.

PART 1
General principles

Assessment of the patient with a squint

This chapter outlines assessment of the squinting patient and includes:

History

Examination

- Orthoptic
  - Assessment of visual acuity
  - Assessment of the deviation
  - Assessment of eye movements
  - Assessment of binocular function
  - Additional tests
- Ophthalmic and medical assessment

Investigation

This chapter aims to emphasize the importance of various tests carried out with regard to the diagnosis, surgical management and prognosis of strabismus.

History

As in all branches of medicine it is vital to have a clear history from the patient regarding all aspects of the strabismus.

Nature of the problem	Cosmesis, diplopia, head posture
Onset of the squint	Acute or gradual. Constant or intermittent. Symptomatic or not
Duration of squint	Childhood or adult life
Course of the squint	Deteriorating, improving or stable
Precipitating factors	Trauma, illness, new glasses, ocular surgery, close or distance work
Relieving factors	Correction of refractive error, sleep, change in head position
Associated symptoms	Diplopia, headache
Past ophthalmic history	Previous surgery, spectacle wear, poor vision in one or both eyes
Risk factors	Family history, birth and developmental history

| Past medical history | Cardiovascular disease, autoimmune disease, endocrine disease, neurological conditions and neurosurgery. Injuries to eye or face |
| Current systematic enquiry | Particular emphasis on cardiovascular, neurological and endocrine symptomatology which may have previously been undiagnosed. Drug history |

These factors should indicate the underlying aetiology of the strabismus and whether the patient has the potential for binocular single vision.

Examination

All those presenting with strabismus require full assessment of the squint and, depending on the nature of the possible diagnosis, may require further examination and investigation.

In the UK many tests regarding strabismus are routinely carried out by orthoptists. Decisions regarding management are, however, made by ophthalmologists and they therefore should be capable of performing orthoptic tests, know the indications for each (Table 1.1), the normal expected findings and ranges and the relevance of an abnormal result with regard to the prognosis of the squint (Table 1.2).

A brief description is given of tests that are important for, but may be unfamiliar to, ophthalmic surgeons. For a full description of other tests (e.g. cover test), an orthoptic text should be consulted.

Assessment of the visual acuity

The visual acuity should be measured in each eye in all patients at every visit. This gives information regarding amblyopia, refractive error and the effect of spectacle wear on the vision.

Surgical treatment should be delayed until the vision is maximized in each eye for those with amblyopia to ensure an optimum result.

- Test each eye separately, using the most appropriate test for age. There are a variety of tests used. The following list is not comprehensive but comprises the tests used by the authors:

Test	Age
Forced choice preferential looking	From birth
Cardiff cards	Age 6 months to 2 years
Kay's pictures	Age 18 months to 3 years
Logmar crowded tests (pictures and letters)	Age 18 months to 5 years (carried out at 3 metres)
Sheridan Gardiner, Sonksten Silver, Cambridge cards	Age 2.5 to 4 years
Sheridan Gardiner with test type	Age 3.5 to 6 years
Snellen chart	Age 4.5 onwards

Table 1.1   Examination of the squinting patient: the role of different tests

All patients
Assessment of visual acuity
Assessment of the deviation – cover test and measurements
Assessment of eye movements – all positions
Binocular function – motor and sensory components
Refraction – cycloplegic in children
Full ophthalmic examination

Accommodative esotropias/distance exotropias
AC/A ratio

Intermittent/latent squints
BVA

Vertical deviations
3 step test
Vertical fusion range

IV nerve palsies
Bielchowsky head tilt test
Vertical fusion range
Amount of torsion

Any paralytic/restrictive
Measurement of deviation – all positions
Hess chart
Field of BSV
Tests of muscle function

Thyroid eye disease
Uniocular fields of fixation
Field of BSV
Vertical fusion range

Patients >8 years with concomitant strabismus
Postoperative diplopia test

Childhood esotropes with good visual acuity
Prism adaptation test

Table 1.2   Importance of investigations regarding the prognosis of a squint

Good prognosis for a functional result
Equal (or nearly equal) visual acuities
No significant reduction in range of movement of the eyes
Evidence of good motor fusion ranges
Evidence of normal sensory binocular function
Lack of suppression

- Patients with nystagmus may have to be tested with both eyes open, or with a plus 10 lens placed in front of the fellow eye in order to test the eyes individually to reduce the effects of latent nystagmus
- Tests involving single letters tend to overestimate the visual acuity in amblyopia and there may be an apparent 'drop' in vision when moving from singles to linear test type. It is therefore always important to note which type of test was used and to progress to linear testing as soon as possible.

Assessment of the deviation

Identification of the squint

It is fundamental that the presence of a squint can be confirmed or refuted on clinical examination, in order to make the diagnosis of strabismus. A squint may be obvious or difficult to detect, particularly in small children. The following tests may be used to detect the presence of a squint:

- Corneal light reflexes – these should be symmetrical. Placed centrally or slightly nasally on each cornea.
- 20 dioptre base out prism test – a 20 dioptre base out prism is placed in front of one eye while the child is fixing on an interesting target. If the child is binocular, the eye will move out to overcome the prism.
- The Brückner test – the patient is examined with a direct ophthalmoscope from about arm's length in a darkened room. The examiner sees a bright red reflex from both eyes when the patient looks in the distance. The patient is then asked to fix on the light of the ophthalmoscope and the red reflex should dim as the pupils constrict. If a squint is present (or if a large refractive error is present) the reflex from the squinting eye will remain bright.
- Cover test – this is the 'gold standard' for the identification of a squint. The cover/uncover test identifies whether a squint is present or not, and whether it is latent or manifest. The alternate cover test identifies the maximum angle of deviation.

The following factors have an influence on the management of the squint:

- the direction of the deviation (horizontal or vertical)
- whether the squint is latent or manifest (and rate of recovery if latent)
- whether it is unilateral or alternating
- whether it is greater for near or distance
- whether it changes in different positions of gaze
- whether it is affected by spectacle wear.

Measurement of the deviation

An accurate, objective measurement of the deviation at each visit identifies the size of the squint, whether there is any change and the effect of any treatment (e.g. glasses or surgery). This is often helpful in deciding when to carry out surgery. The amount of surgery performed is strongly influenced by the size of the deviation. Measurements are required:

- for near and distance deviations in all cases (for horizontal and vertical deviations)
- for upgaze and downgaze in vertical squints
- in lateral gaze for exotropias to measure any lateral incomitance
- in all 9 positions of gaze in incomitant squints
- for the degree of torsion in patients with IV nerve palsies.

METHODS

- The prism cover test is the most accurate method of measuring the angle of squint, and should be carried out in all cases if possible. Uncooperative patients and those with blind eyes or eccentric fixation may be assessed by less accurate methods.
  - Corneal reflections (Hirschberg), which estimate the size of a squint by using the position of the corneal reflection on the deviating eye (approximately 30 dioptres if the reflex is at the pupil margin, 45 dioptres if it is mid-way between the pupil margin and the limbus and 60 dioptres if it is at the limbus).
  - The prism reflection test (Krimsky), which uses prisms to centre the corneal reflection of the squinting eye.
- The synoptophore is useful in those with large angled deviations and for measuring the deviation in all 9 positions of gaze.

Cyclotorsion

The presence of torsion can help to differentiate between congenital and acquired IV nerve palsies (torsion is not appreciated in congenital cases) and between unilateral and bilateral IV nerve palsies. When considering surgical management, torsion may be a significant barrier to regaining binocular single vision and needs to be taken into account when formulating a surgical plan.

Torsion can be tested using:

- double Maddox rods
- the synoptophore – using dedicated torsion slides
- fundoscopy
- the Lees screen – using the tiltometer adaptation
- the torsionometer.

Assessment of the eye movements

The accurate assessment of eye movements is essential in reaching a diagnosis of the squinting patient. Any abnormality in any direction should be identified. Movements should be recorded in a manner that is sensitive to changes in muscle function, as decisions about surgery may be dependent on the stability of certain movements. The surgical procedure performed is highly dependent upon the pattern of incomitance.

- The eyes should be examined in all 9 positions of gaze and also in convergence.
- Any change in the angle of squint is observed and confirmed using the cover test (and measured using the prism cover test where indicated).
- Any pattern of weakness, overaction or restriction of muscles is noted.
- A or V patterns should be noted by observing change in the horizontal deviation on upgaze and downgaze.
- The presence and magnitude of any nystagmus should be noted in different directions of gaze.
- It may be necessary to test the movements for distance as well as for near (e.g. in suspected VI nerve palsies) and this can be done by asking the patient to fixate a distance target and move the head around.

The standard method of assessing eye movements is to test pursuit movements by asking the patient to follow a slowly moving target with both eyes, comparing the versions in all positions of gaze. Vergence movements (convergence and divergence) are also tested. If a reduction in movement is suspected or identified, then monocular duction testing should be performed, testing each eye in turn, while the other eye is covered. This is helpful in confirming the reduction in movement.

In those with neurological disease or deficit then more complex examination may be required, including testing rapid eye movements (saccades), optokinetic movements and doll's head responses.

Charting eye movements

The Hess (or Lees) chart is a useful method of evaluating eye movements and provides a record of the stability, improvement or deterioration in those with incomitant deviations. The eyes are fully dissociated for this test, which depends on Hering's and Sherington's laws.

- This chart assesses the central area (out to 30 degrees), so deviations at extremes of gaze may not be represented on it.
- The movement of one eye is compared with that of the other (which makes it less useful in those with bilateral disease, e.g. symmetrical cases of thyroid eye disease).
- Patients must have simultaneous perception (normal or abnormal retinal correspondence) in order to perform this test.

- It is useful for adults, but cannot be used for children under 8 years of age as they are unable to cooperate sufficiently.

Uniocular field of fixation (UFOF) is an objective method of charting the extent of ductions of each eye individually, using a perimeter. It is principally used to monitor the progress of eye movements in thyroid eye disease.

Field of binocular single vision (BSV) is a chart of the area of the visual field over which the patient can achieve binocular single vision. It measures the limits of conjugate movement through which single vision is maintained. It is useful in monitoring the progression or recovery of an acquired motility defect such as a blow out fracture, nerve palsy or thyroid eye disease. It is helpful in deciding when to operate in such cases as treatment is aimed at restoring a useful field of BSV. It is useful for medico-legal purposes (it can be scored to quantify disability of reduced field).

Assessment of binocular function

The assessment of a patient's binocular function is necessary in order to determine whether they do or do not have the potential for binocular single vision. Binocular single vision may be normal, reflecting bifoveal fixation, or abnormal, when the fovea from one eye shares an extra-foveal corresponding retinal point with the other eye (as seen in patients with microtropia). Patients who demonstrate constant suppression do not have binocular single vision. Knowledge about binocular function is vital in understanding the aetiology of the strabismus, planning the management and providing a prognosis for treatment.

The state of retinal correspondence

Knowledge regarding the state of retinal correspondence is important as this indicates whether the patient has potential for normal binocular vision, abnormal binocular vision or no potential for binocular vision at all. Tests used to investigate this include:

- Bagolini striated glasses
- Worth's four dot test – red and green light
- The synoptophore using simultaneous perception slides (dissimilar images on each slide)
- The 4 dioptre prism test – this test is used to assess the presence or absence of bifoveal fixation and is useful in diagnosing the presence of a microtropia/central foveal suppression scotoma in small angled squints or in those with small inequalities in vision.

Fusion

Fusion has two components – sensory and motor fusion.

SENSORY FUSION

Sensory fusion is the ability to perceive two similar images, one with each eye and to interpret them as one. This can be either:

- central, reflecting bifoveal fixation (as seen in those with normal binocular single vision) or
- peripheral, reflecting peripheral fixation (as seen in those with abnormal binocular single vision).

Tests used to investigate this include:

- Worth's 4 dot test – red and green lights
- Synoptophore using superimposition slides.

MOTOR FUSION

Motor fusion is the component of binocular vision that maintains visual alignment of the eyes through a range of vergences.

There are four main components of motor fusion:

- positive fusional vergence (convergence)
- negative fusional vergence (divergence)
- vertical fusion
- cyclovergence.

Knowledge of the patient's fusional amplitudes gives information regarding the ability or potential ability to control a deviation. Poor or reduced motor fusion is a bad prognostic feature regarding the success of squint surgery, even in the presence of excellent sensory function (i.e. high grade stereopsis). A clear knowledge of both the motor and sensory elements of binocular function is essential.

Motor fusion can be evaluated using:

- The horizontal fusion range, which indicates the power of horizontal motor fusion using a horizontal prism bar and a target. The synoptophore can also be used and has the advantage of allowing for correction of the deviation prior to the measurement of motor fusion. The test should be performed at near and distance and the positive (or base out) horizontal fusion range measures up to 35–40 dioptres at near (15 dioptres at distance). The negative or (base in) fusion range – up to 10 dioptres for near (and less for distance, 4–6 dioptres).
- The 20 dioptre prism test gives an indication whether motor fusion is present (usually used in young children). It is not quantitative, but simply indicates that the child has diplopia induced by the prism and has the fusional ability to overcome this.
- Binocular visual acuity (BVA) gives a measure of the strength of motor fusion, which indicates degree of control of a latent or intermittent deviation. This is helpful in deciding whether a squint is breaking down and hence when to operate, particularly in patients with intermittent or latent deviations. (See earlier, Assessment of the Deviation.)

- Ask the patient to read from the top of the Snellen chart (or equivalent)
- Perform the alternate cover test as they read down the chart, ensuring complete dissociation
- At each line allow the patient to regain binocular viewing
- The measurement is taken when they no longer can recover to binocular vision to read the letters
- The BVA should be as good as the visual acuity of the less good eye
- A large vertical fusion range suggests a long-standing or slowly developing condition, e.g. thyroid eye disease or congenital IV nerve palsy. When planning surgery, the presence of an extended range indicates that the aim of surgery should be an undercorrection of the deviation. The normal range is up to 3 dioptres up or down.

Stereopsis

Stereopsis is the perception of depth based on binocular disparity and comes in two forms:

- high grade, which is associated with central fusion (60 seconds of arc or better)
- peripheral, which is associated with peripheral fusion.

Tests of stereopsis can be qualitative or quantitative (measured in seconds of arc).

- Frisby
- Titmus/Wirt
- Randot, TNO
- Lang
- Synoptophore.

Suppression

Suppression is usually acquired in childhood whereas adults who acquire a strabismus usually develop diplopia as they cannot suppress. In some instances suppression can be lost – spontaneously, following injury or surgery. Tests for the presence of suppression include:

- Bagolini glasses
- Worth's lights
- The 4 dioptre prism test is used to diagnose central suppression and is useful in diagnosing microtropia.

Additional tests

Having carried out these tests, a provisional diagnosis should be possible, but additional measurements or assessment may be required in order to confirm the findings or in order to prepare for surgery.

Postoperative diplopia test

This test identifies whether a patient is at risk of developing postoperative diplopia by using prisms to optically simulate the surgical correction. A base out prism bar is placed in front of the deviating eye in esotropia, gradually increasing the strength until the patient is slightly overcorrected, in order to identify whether diplopia is experienced within the angle that would be surgically corrected. Base in prisms are used in the same way for exotropia. This is used in patients who have suppression and are being considered for cosmetic surgery to improve the angle of deviation. If it indicates that there is a risk of double vision the patient should have a diagnostic injection of botulinum toxin before considering surgical correction (see Chapter 15).

AC/A ratio

This is the amount of accommodative convergence induced by accommodation (measured in prism dioptres). This ratio is inborn in each individual and remains the same throughout life, unless changed by surgery. Some individuals exert an excessive amount of accommodative convergence (a high AC/A ratio) and this has a role in the development of strabismus and also has an influence on management.

It is vital to know the AC/A ratio in those with convergence excess esotropia and those with distance exotropia in making the definitive diagnosis and formulating a management plan. There are two methods of measuring AC/A ratio in common usage, the gradient method, which is the easier and more accurate method and the heterophoria method.

The normal range is 3.5–5/1.

Prism adaptation test

Some children with esotropia manifest only a proportion of their full angle of squint and if they are corrected either with prisms or surgery they will increase to this full angle. Preoperative prism adaptation helps to diagnose the maximum angle of deviation and the potential for a binocular result in these children. It is most useful in those who, on testing, can be shown to demonstrate peripheral fusion at an angle greater than their angle of deviation. These patients would be undercorrected surgically if they were not prism adapted and the amount of surgery is therefore correspondingly increased. It is therefore important to know the full angle of squint before surgical intervention. It is only useful in those with good vision in both eyes (>6/18) and in those with relatively small angled squints (35 dioptres or less).

This is assessed by placing Fresnel prisms to correct the deviation in front of one or both eyes for a few days in order to ensure the full size of the deviation is realized and to identify whether a binocular result is to be expected.

Three step test

This test assists in the diagnosis of vertical muscle weakness in all patients with a vertical squint. It is essential in those suspected of having a superior oblique palsy to differentiate this from a contra-lateral superior rectus palsy and to help to detect bilateral IV nerve palsy.

- Step 1: which eye is hypertropic?
  A cover test identifies this. The elevators of the low eye (inferior oblique or superior rectus) are affected or the depressors of the high eye (superior oblique or inferior rectus) are affected.
- Step 2: is the hypertropia greater in right or left gaze?
  If the height increases when the eyes move away from the high eye this narrows down the possible weak muscle to either the superior oblique of the adducted eye (superior oblique depresses the eye in adduction) or a contralateral superior rectus weakness (superior rectus elevates the eye in abduction). Conversely if the height increases when the eyes move in the direction of the higher eye this suggests either weak inferior rectus of the abducted eye (inferior rectus depresses the eye in abduction) or weak inferior oblique of the adducted eye (inferior oblique elevates the eye in adduction) – this is much rarer.
- Step 3: is the hypertropia larger on elevation or depression to the affected side?
  A cover test is performed in upgaze and downgaze to the side that has the maximum deviation. This identifies which of the contralateral muscles is responsible for the vertical deviation.

Bielchowsky head tilt test

This test helps to identify a superior oblique weakness. When the head is tilted to the right the right eye intorts (and the left eye extorts). The intorters of the eye are the superior oblique and the superior rectus – their vertical pulls cancelling one another out if both are healthy. If the superior oblique is weak, however, the relatively unopposed superior rectus causes a hypertropia (or an increased hypertropia) to develop in the intorting eye. This should be performed in all vertical squints where the diagnosis is not known.

Tests of muscle function

These tests are used in cases of incomitant strabismus to help to differentiate between weakness and restriction of muscles (IOP and forced duction) or between paresis and palsy (force generation). This is information that is necessary as the surgical approach to each possibility is vastly different.

DIFFERENTIAL IOP READINGS IN DIFFERENT POSITIONS OF GAZE

- The IOP goes up when a tight muscle pushes against the globe.
- Tight IR on elevation leads to increased IOP in upgaze.
- An increase of 5 mmHg or more indicates some degree of inferior rectus tightness (often it is 10–20 mmHg more).

FORCED DUCTION TEST

This can be carried out under general or topical anaesthesia.

- When performed under *general anaesthesia* this is usually before commencing strabismus surgery. It is also useful during surgery to test the effects of moving the position of muscle.
    - Grasp the conjunctiva with two pairs of toothed forceps that are applied at opposite sides of the limbus and attempt to move the eye as far as possible
        - if this is possible the muscle is weak
        - if it is not then there is restriction.
    - To test the rectus muscles pull the eye forward as this is carried out.
    - To test the obliques, push the eye backwards into the orbit.

- Using topical anaesthesia

    - Most adults can cooperate with this test, but it is not suitable for children.
    - Instill plenty of topical anaesthetic with a cotton bud soaked in anaesthetic over the area to be grasped.
    - Close the eye not being examined.
    - Ask the patient to look as far as they can in the direction of the 'weak' muscle.
    - Grasp the anaesthetized conjunctiva with toothed forceps and attempt to move the eye further than the patient can.

FORCE GENERATION TEST

Used to differentiate muscle paresis from palsy.

- This requires patient cooperation and therefore cannot be carried out under general anaesthesia.
- Topical anaesthetic is applied to the conjunctiva.
- The patient is asked to look as far as they can in the direction of the weak muscle.
- The anaesthetized conjunctiva is grasped with toothed forceps at the limbus opposite the muscle being tested and it is attempted to move the eye in the opposite direction in order to test the resistance
    - if this is possible with no resistance the muscle is completely palsied
    - if this is possible but some resistance is encountered the muscle is partially palsied (or paretic).

Refraction

All patients with strabismus should be fully refracted. This will detect some of the causes of secondary strabismus and determine the role of spectacles in the possible aetiology and management of the squint.

- In the case of children this should always be a full cycloplegic refraction (adults in whom there may be an accommodative element to their strabismus also require this).
- Cyclopentolate 1% drops are instilled twice (5 minutes apart) into each eye.
- The full hypermetropic correction should be prescribed (minus working distance only) in all children who have esotropia.
- Atropine refraction is useful in those who still have esotropia despite being in a full refraction following a cyclopentolate refraction. Instill atropine 1% drops twice a day for 3 days and on the morning of the refraction to ensure a full effect.

A full ophthalmic examination

All patients presenting with strabismus should have a full ophthalmic examination to identify any potential causes or risk factors for primary or secondary strabismus and any associated abnormalities that may influence management.

- External examination – facial appearance, lid position, orbital anatomy, epicanthus.
- Slit lamp examination – scleral/conjunctival scars from previous squint surgery, iris atrophy (albinism may be very subtle), cataract.
- Pupil reactions – afferent or efferent reactions, equality of size.
- Dilated fundoscopy – optic nerve head, macula, clarity of media, retinal periphery.
- Fields of vision – in patients with neurological deficit or extensive glaucoma.

Examination and investigation for systemic disease

The majority of patients with strabismus require no systemic examination or investigation, however, in a few cases this is required to exclude or confirm underlying systemic disease.

Clinical examination

A full medical and neurological examination should be performed before investigating patients with nerve palsies. Patients with possible thyroid eye disease should be examined for other clinical features of thyroid dysfunction. Those with suspected myasthenia gravis should be fatigued, for evidence of increasing problems. Patients with blow out fractures should be examined for other features of facial trauma.

Investigations for microvascular disease (nerve palsies)

- Blood pressure – hypertension.
- Urinalysis – diabetes.
- Blood investigations – full blood count, plasma viscosity, triglycerides and cholesterol, fasting or random blood glucose.

Thyroid disease

Thyroid function tests, thyroid antibodies.

Myasthenia gravis

- Tensilon test.
- Trial of pyridostigmine. (Acetyl-choline receptor antibodies are not commonly positive in ocular myasthenia and are expensive!)

Radiological investigations

CT scan: CT scans are excellent at demonstrating orbital anatomy and are particularly useful when looking for bony anomalies, such as blow out fractures.

MRI: MRI is particularly good at delineating soft tissues, but does not show bone.
This is the best investigation for possible brain-stem lesions (for III, IV or VI lesions) or lesions along the optic pathways. Orbital MRI can be enhanced by the use of a surface coil. The short tau inverse recovery (STIR) sequence gives excellent detail of the optic nerve and is useful for those with possible thyroid eye disease or active orbital lesions. Rectus muscle oedema can be estimated with MRI scanning and hence is useful in identifying the degree of orbital inflammation.

MRA: Magnetic resonance angiography is useful in detecting suspected intracranial aneurysms, useful in painful third nerve palsies.

Further reading

Ansons AM, Davis H. *Diagnosis and management of ocular motility disorders.* Blackwell Science, Oxford. 2001

Aylward GW, McCarry B, Kousoulides L, Lee JP, Fells P. A scoring method of Hess charts. *Eye* 1992; **6**: 659–61

Fitzsimmons R, White JS. Functional scoring of the field of binocular vision. *Ophthalmology* 1990; **97**: 33–5

Gray C, Ansons A, Spencer A. The method of testing and recording of the post-operative diplopia test. *Br Orthoptic J* 1996; **53**: 51

Krimsky E. The binocular examination of the young child. *Am J Ophthalmol* 1943; **26**: 624

Mayer L, Fulton A, Rodier D. Grating and recognition acuities of pediatric patients. *Ophthalmology* 1984; **91**: 947

Mein J, Moore S. (eds) The evaluation of the Bielchowsky head tilt test. In: *Orthoptics, research and practice*, Kimpton, London. 1981; 189

Pratt-Johnson JA, Tilson G. *Management of strabismus and amblyopia: a practical guide*. Theime Medical Publishers, New York. 1994

Prism Adaptation Study Research Group. Efficacy of prism adaptation in the surgical management of acquired esotropia. *Arch Ophthalmol* 1990; **108**: 1248–56

Rowe FJ. *Clinical orthoptics*. Blackwell Science, Oxford. 1997

Sloan L, Sears ML, Jablonski MD. Convergence-accommodation relationships. *Arch Ophthalmol* 1960; **63**: 283

Von Noorden GK. *Binocular vision and ocular motility; theory and management of strabismus*, 5th edn. CV Mosby Co., St Louis. 1996

2

Non-surgical management of strabismus

> The forms of non-surgical management considered in this chapter are:
>
> **Optical treatment**
>
> **Prisms**
>
> **Orthoptic exercises**
>
> **Eye drops**
>
> **Amblyopia treatment**
>
> **Treatment of insuperable diplopia**
>
> **Botulinum toxin**

Although this text is primarily aimed at the surgical management of strabismus, this chapter briefly examines non-surgical methods of treating strabismus. They need to be understood to ensure that surgery is used appropriately. They may also be required to prepare patients for surgery or to consolidate a surgical result. The various forms of non-surgical management are often used in conjunction with surgical treatment.

Indications

Non-surgical methods of strabismus management can be used:

- as definitive treatment – in many instances surgery is not indicated – e.g. fully accommodative esotropia, convergence insufficiency
- in order to prepare for surgery – e.g. amblyopia treatment
- as an interim, until stable enough for surgery – e.g. prisms or occlusion to deal with diplopia until it is clear that there are no further changes in an evolving or recovering strabismus
- as an alternative to surgery in those who are not well enough for, or do not wish, surgical treatment
- as an alternative to surgery in those with little chance of surgical success – e.g. in some complex motility disorders such as following

significant orbital trauma or complete third nerve palsy as a satisfactory outcome is unlikely due to motor factors

- in those with insuperable diplopia (i.e. who have lost all binocular function and also have no suppression areas) or those with insufficient field to support binocular vision (e.g. tunnel vision, severe bitemporal hemianopias) as a satisfactory outcome is not possible due to sensory factors.

Methods

a) Optical treatment
b) Prisms
c) Orthoptic exercises
d) Eye drops
e) Amblyopia treatment
f) Treatment of insuperable diplopia
g) Botulinum toxin

a) *Optical treatment of refractive errors and the prescription of glasses*

i) Indications for spectacle correction

- The need to relieve accommodation and therefore help control esotropia.
- The need to prevent amblyopia developing in an eye(s) that sees poorly for refractive reasons.
- The need to improve a child's vision, as poor visual acuity in one or both eyes can be a barrier to the development of binocular function.

All patients with strabismus should have refraction performed, including adults. In children a cycloplegic refraction is required, usually using cyclopentolate drops 1% instilled twice in a period of 5 minutes. Those with very dark irides or who appear to have residual accommodation despite the full optical correction may require atropine 1% instead. This is usually given twice daily for 3 days prior to and on the morning of the day of the appointment for refraction.

PRESCRIPTION OF HYPERMETROPIA

Any hypermetropic correction should be given to children with convergent strabismus. The full retinoscopic findings are prescribed – taking only the working distance away with no reduction in the prescription for the cycloplegia. Uncorrected hypermetropia of +4.00 or more carries a high risk of bilateral amblyopia and should be corrected in all children.

PRESCRIPTION OF MYOPIA

Myopia is relatively uncommon in young children. Full correction, even low levels, should be prescribed in children with exotropia. A child of school age with myopia requires a prescription for glasses, but under this age children rarely present with myopia as they are usually asymptomatic. In all cases the weakest prescription with which the child can see should be prescribed.

ANISOMETROPIA

The squinting eye is usually the eye with the larger refractive error and, if this is not the case, examine the eyes carefully for retinal or optic nerve problems and/or check the refraction and the effect of the cycloplegia. When prescribing glasses, always prescribe the full difference between the two eyes. If there is no squint, anisometropia of more than 1.00 dioptres is an indication for glasses, to prevent the development of amblyopia.

ASTIGMATISM

Children with significant astigmatism are at risk of developing amblyopia. Any cylindrical correction of >1.5 dioptres which is persistent (as astigmatism may diminish rapidly) should be corrected.

EFFECT ON EYE GROWTH

Correction of hypermetropia with glasses may retard normal emmetropization in childhood and so should not be carried out routinely unless there is an indication (see below). Conversely, there is no evidence that correction of myopia has any effect on the rate of progression of the myopia and, to date, there is no treatment that has yet been demonstrated to prevent or retard the progression of myopia.

Table 2.1 summarizes glasses prescription for children between the ages of 12 months and 5 years. All measurements of the refraction are after the working distance has been taken into account. 'High-risk' of developing a squint exists if there is a strong family history, or if an intermittent squint has been observed.

Spectacles are the mainstay of optical treatment. Contact lenses are rarely used in children, although they are very useful for high degrees of ametropia. Permanent correction of hypermetropia by excimer laser

Table 2.1   Refractive correction of children – 1–5 years

	No squint	*Convergent squint*	*Divergent squint*	*High-risk of squint*
Hypermetropia	Prescribe if > +4.00	Prescribe *all* plus	Prescribe if > +4.00	Prescribe if > +2.00
Myopia	Prescribe if symptoms (or > −3)	Prescribe if symptoms (or > −3)	Prescribe all minus	Prescribe if symptoms (or > −3)
Anisometropia	Prescribe if > or = +1.0 difference	Prescribe all plus	Prescribe all minus	Prescribe if > or = +1.0 difference

treatment should not be used in children since the long-term effects on a developing eye are not known and the technique is not yet reliable enough in treating hypermetropes.

ii) Bifocal glasses are used in patients who have a covergence excess esotropia, due to a high A/C:A ratio

The lower segment lenses reduce the need to accommodate and therefore reduce the angle of squint for near.

- Children should be given the lowest reading addition that allows them to maintain binocular single vision for close work.
- Bifocals are most suitable for children who are able to read, as younger children tend not to use the bifocal segment.
- Bifocals for children should always be fitted very carefully and they must be of the 'executive' type, with the lower segment set high to bisect the optic axis horizontally. If these are not dispensed the child will look over the top of the lens for close work.

This form of treatment is not always acceptable to the affected child, or their parents. In addition they work by suspending accommodation fully and therefore may have long-term effects associated with hypo-accommodation. For these reasons most ophthalmologists in the UK prefer surgical management of patients with near esotropia, although they may be useful in such patients while they are awaiting surgery, those with residual strabismus following surgery or those who do not wish to undergo or are unsuitable for surgery.

iii) Decentration of spectacle lenses

Patients with a large compensatory head posture who have a significant refractive error may benefit from decentration of their spectacle lenses. This allows the patient to look through the optical centre of their spectacles and improve the visual acuity.

iv) Fogging

In patients with DVD which predominantly affects one eye it may be possible to promote fixation with the affected eye by fogging the other eye by increasing or reducing the spectacle prescription.

b) Prisms

Prisms are placed in front of the eye with the apex pointing towards the direction of the deviation:

- base in for exodeviations
- base out for esodeviations
- base down for hyperdeviations

- base up for hypodeviations
- prisms *cannot* correct torsional diplopia.

Prisms may be used temporarily or permanently in the management of squint.

- Temporary use of prisms involves placing a plastic, stick on (or Fresnel) prism over the lens of spectacles. Plano glasses can be used for those who do not wear a correction. The prism will reduce the visual acuity slightly and this may be significant with large prisms. Stick on plastic prisms are useful for:
    - Relief of symptomatic diplopia by restoring binocular vision, while awaiting spontaneous recovery (e.g. nerve palsies) or surgery
    - Promotion of binocular function in children with potential binocular vision (e.g. acute VI nerve palsies or overcorrection of an intermittent exotropia)
- Long-term use of prisms involves the incorporation of prisms into the spectacle lens
    - Patients who are unfit for or unwilling to undergo surgical correction
    - Small angled squints with diplopia, for symptomatic relief.

The smallest size of prism that makes the patient comfortable should be used. For practical purposes prisms are not usually used for large deviations. Prisms are less useful in patients with incomitant squints, as the angle of deviation varies in different positions of gaze. Patients with decompensating heterophoria may gradually require more and more prism to control the deviation.

c) Orthoptic exercises

Some types of squint respond well to orthoptic exercises. They may be used to treat symptoms associated with strabismus: to aid control or to promote improvement in sensory or motor function so that the results of surgery are optimized. Orthoptic treatment should be carried out under the careful supervision of experienced orthoptists with clear aims and objectives in each case. Inappropriate use of orthoptic exercises may lead to the development of insuperable diplopia. Methods of treatment are outwith the remit of this text, but include:

- improving fusional amplitudes to improve control of a squint (used in intermittent deviations and decompensating phorias)
- teaching recognition of diplopia in order to help to control a deviation (used in fully accommodative esotropias)
- anti-supppression treatment (used in convergence insufficiency and intermittent strabismus – in order to teach control of the deviation)
- improving near point of convergence (used in convergence insufficiency).

d) Eye drops

Miotic and cycloplegic eye drops can be used to modify or treat strabismus.

- Miotics
  - These drops reduce the need to accommodate and are useful in the diagnosis and treatment of convergence excess (high AC/A ratio). They are used in both eyes.
    ○ Phospholine iodide (PI), now unavailable in this country except on a named patient basis, has the advantage of once daily instillation, but has a number of significant side effects
    ○ Pilocarpine is used, but requires frequent instillation and is less effective than PI
  - These are not recommended for long-term treatment as they do not offer a long-term cure
- Cycloplegics
  - Atropine or cyclopentolate can be used to promote spectacle wear in children who have difficulty relaxing their accommodation. They are only required for 1–2 weeks
  - Cycloplegics can also be used as a form of occlusion (see below).

e) Amblyopia treatment

Patients with amblyopia require treatment to improve the visual acuity in the eye(s) with reduced vision. Treatment should take place during the 'sensitive period' of development, i.e. less than 8 years of age. It should be carried out under the supervision of an orthoptist, with regular review and testing of the vision in both eyes. Ideally treatment should take place until the vision in both eyes is equal, but this is not always achievable and the optimum vision has to be accepted.

Treatment options include:

- Correction of refractive error – visual acuity in children with ametropic amblyopia often responds to wear of the correct spectacle prescription with no further intervention required
- Occlusion – the normal eye is covered, usually with a patch, to stimulate the other eye. This should always be carried out with spectacle correction in place, if a refractive error is present
- Cycloplegic drops – are useful in children who do not cooperate with patching as they cannot 'cheat' so easily. Atropine 1% drops are instilled daily into the preferred fixing eye. This is only useful in mild to moderate degrees of amblyopia. It has a particular role in patients with latent nystagmus.
- Penalization – the vision in the better eye is reduced by instilling cycloplegic drops. This can be further refined by enhancing the vision in the amblyopic eye for near with the use of a plus lens to this eye (near penalization).

f) Treatments for insuperable diplopia

It is not always possible to restore either binocular vision or a useful area of suppression to relieve diplopia. In such cases reduction of vision in the squinting eye is usually considered. Patients vary in their ability to ignore the diplopia and some may require complete occlusion in order to achieve this. This can be achieved by:

- occlusive patches worn over the squinting eye – usually placed over the spectacle lens to protect the skin around the eye
- occlusive lenses in the glasses – these may also be used mask extremely unsightly squints, but neutral density filter lenses may be as effective, but less obvious
- occlusive contact lens – in the form of a painted contact lens
- occlusive intraocular lens – care must be taken to ensure that the IOL is larger than the pupil, which may be dilated in cases of trauma or III nerve palsy.

The former two options are commonly used in the short term and the latter possibilities are more useful as a longer-term solutions.

g) Botulinum toxin

Botulinum toxin is a tool that can be used diagnostically to formulate a management plan for patients with strabismus, or therapeutically to treat patients either alone or in combination with surgery (see Chapter 15 for details).

Further reading

Albert DG, Hiles DA. Myopia, bifocals and accommodation. *Am Orthoptic J* 1969; **19**: 59

Ansons AM, Davis H. *Diagnosis and management of ocular motility disorders.* Chapter 8 Non surgical management. Blackwell Science, Oxford. 2001

Blakemore C, Cooper G. Development of the brain depends on the visual environment. *Nature* 1970; **228**: 477

Campos EC. Review of amblyopia. *Surv Ophthalmol* 1994; **40**: 23

Dorey F, Adams GG, Lee JP, Sloper JJ. Intensive occlusion treatment for amblyopia. *Br J Ophthalmol* 200; **85**: 310–3

Goldstein JH. The role of miotics in strabismus. *Surv Ophthalmol* 1968; **13**: 31

Gregersen E, Pontoppodian M, Rindziunski E. Optic and drug penalization and favouring in the treatment of squinting amblyopia. *Acta Ophthalmol* 1965; **43**: 462

Hubel DH, Wiesel TN. Laminar and columnar distribution of geniculo-cortical fibres in the Macaque monkey. *J Comparative Neurol* 1972; **146**: 421

Ludwig IL, Parks MM, Jetson PP. Long-term results of bifocal therapy for accommodative esotropia. *J Pediatr Ophthalmol Strabismus* 1989; **26**: 264

Lymburn E, Malik TY, MacEwen CJ. Dioptre for dioptre. Is there a relationship between the refractive error and the angle of squint? *Br Orthoptic J* 2000; **57**: 23–7

Luke NE. Antisuppression exercises in exodeviations. *Am Orthoptic J* 1970; **20**: 100

Montes-Mico R. Astigmatism in infancy and childhood. *J Pediatr Ophthalmol Strabismus* 2000; **37**: 349–53

Repka MX, Ray JM. The efficacy of optical and pharmacological penalization. *Ophthalmology* 1993; **100**: 769

Rowe FJ. *Clinical orthoptics*. Blackwell Science, Oxford. 1997

Sandy CJ, Wilson S, Brian Page A, Frazer DG, McGinnity FG, Lee JP. Phacoemulsification and opaque intraocular lens implantation for the treatment of intractable diplopia. *Ophthalmic Surg Lasers* 2000; **31**: 429–31

Veronneau-Troutman S. Fresnel prism membrane in the treatment of strabismus. *Can J Ophthalmol* 1971; **6**: 249

von Noorden GK, Morris J, Edelman P. Efficacy of bifocals in the treatment of accommodative esotropia. *Am J Ophthalmol* 1978; **85**: 830

von Noorden GK. Amblyopia, a multi-disciplinary approach. *Invest Ophthalmol Vis Sci* 1985; **26**: 1704

3

Principles of the surgical management of strabismus

This chapter deals with:

Indications for surgical treatment of strabismus

Timing of surgery

Principles of surgical treatment

Sutures

Anaesthesia for strabismus surgery

Indications for surgical treatment of squint

The indications for squint surgery fall into two categories, functional or cosmetic.

1. Functional: to straighten the eyes with the aim of using both eyes as a single unit
- Alignment of the eyes to promote or restore the development of binocular single vision in children
- Re-alignment of the eyes in patients who had established binocular single vision. Such patients commonly have diplopia and the aim is to restore single vision.

2. Cosmetic: to place the eyes in a cosmetically pleasing position, but with no possibility of gaining binocular vision
- Patients who have a manifest squint with established suppression
- Eyes that have a strabismus in a blind eye
- Patients with diplopia in all directions of gaze, whether the squint is corrected or not, with no area of suppression

In all cosmetic cases, careful preoperative assessment must be carried out to ensure that double vision will not be induced or made worse by surgery.

Timing of surgery

Children

It is important that any amblyopia is treated prior to squint surgery for children and that the parents are aware that this treatment may need to be continued after the operation.

Functional

- To promote binocular vision: the timing of squint surgery is determined by the requirements to promote the development of binocular vision. If early-onset esotropia is treated surgically at an early stage, there is a chance that some degree of binocular vision may develop (usually peripheral fusion).
- To restore binocular vision: if a squint occurs in a child who has already developed binocular vision (e.g. decompensated squints or acquired nerve palsies) then surgery should be performed as soon as the strabismus is stable so that binocular function is not lost. Occlusion may be required to prevent amblyopia in young children.

Cosmetic

- In cases where there is no binocular vision, surgical treatment can be performed at any time, dependent upon the wishes of the parents and the child, although this is often carried out before the child starts school. Surgery should be postponed until amblyopia treatment is complete. Postponing any cosmetic surgery until the child is older allows them to have some input into the decision making, if this is considered appropriate.

Adults

Functional

- Decompensated phorias – treatment should be carried out as soon as reasonably possible to reduce the patient's symptoms and to ensure that suppression does not develop.
- Surgery for acquired pathology should be postponed until the disease process has stabilized. For example, in thyroid eye disease, surgery should not be performed until the inflammatory phase of the condition has passed; in cases of acute nerve palsy, surgery should not be performed until there has been ample time for spontaneous resolution – usually about 6 months.

Cosmetic

- In adults, cosmetic squint surgery can be performed at any time.

Principles of surgical management

Surgical treatment of squint involves altering the relative strengths of the extraocular muscles to realign the eyes. This is done by weakening or strengthening specific muscles, based upon measurements made pre-operatively, the type of squint, the pattern of eye movements, the age of the patient and the aims of treatment. These measurements should include assessment of the squint in the direction of action of any muscle that is to be operated upon, e.g. measurements in downgaze with inferior rectus surgery.

A weakening procedure is always preferable to a strengthening procedure and should be performed if possible. When weakening and strengthening ipsilateral antagonists, surgery should be performed on the muscle to be weakened first.

Which eye?/which muscle?

The decision regarding which muscle(s) to operate on may, or may not, be obvious.

- In a concomitant squint there is no extraocular muscle abnormality and the balance between the eyes needs to be altered
  - It is possible to operate on either or both eyes
  - In practice, surgery tends to be directed to the eye which is amblyopic, or more commonly squinting, as patients perceive this to be the 'squinting eye'
  - Surgery to the medial and lateral rectus muscles of the same eye is common if there is no or little disparity between the angle of squint for near and distance
  - Symmetrical medial rectus surgery is favoured in squints that occur predominately for near, and lateral rectus surgery for distance, deviations
- In patients with muscle restrictions, e.g. tight inferior rectus muscles due to thyroid eye disease, then it is obvious which muscle(s) have to be weakened
- When a muscle is weak, treating over-action of the ipsilateral antagonist to improve movements of that eye, followed by weakening the contralateral synergist to improve the field of BSV is the preferred order of surgery.

Methods of weakening muscles

- *Recession:* this weakens a muscle by placing the insertion further back on the globe and therefore effectively reducing the distance between the origin and insertion of the muscle (Figures 12.1–12.4 and 13.2). Recession should not place the insertion of the muscle behind the equator.
- *Disinsertion* (myotomy/tenotomy): all or part of the insertion of the

muscle is cut free, allowing it to retract and make a new, more recessed attachment to the globe. In muscular muscles this is a myotomy, in tendinous muscles this is called a tenotomy. This must be used with care as it is less controlled than a recession. It is commonly used for the inferior oblique (Figure 13.1) or for superior oblique (often just the posterior or depressing portion, although can be total in certain cases – Figures 13.5 and 13.6). Full myotomy is not used to weaken the rectus muscles but, with care, a central myotomy, which involves releasing the central portion of the muscle from its insertion, but leaving the peripheral parts attached, can be effective when a muscle has already been maximally recessed.

- *Faden:* a suture is placed through the belly of the muscle and it is attached to the sclera at the equator of the eye (Figure 12.8). This weakens the muscle progressively as it moves into its field of action and does not affect the position of the eye in the primary position.

Methods of strengthening muscles

- *Resection:* the muscle is strengthened by cutting a measured amount out of the muscle and placing the new end at the original insertion, which makes the muscle effectively shorter and tighter (Figure 12.5).
- *Advancement:* the insertion of the muscle is moved forward to make the distance between the origin and the insertion further apart (Figure 12.6). This is mostly used in muscles that have been previously recessed, returning them to their original insertion. It causes unsightly scarring if the muscles are brought too far forward towards the limbus.

  - *Harado-Ito:* the original Harada-Ito procedure was the placement of a deviating suture in the anterior fibres of the superior oblique tendon. Fells modification of this is a type of advancement that is performed only on the anterior portion of the superior oblique tendon, advancing it along its field of action towards the superior border of the lateral rectus (Figure 13.7). The original procedure is now rarely performed.

- *Tuck:* instead of cutting a piece out of a muscle, the muscle is shortened by folding over (or tucking) a portion of the muscle (Figure 13.4). This is really only used for the superior oblique tendon as other muscles are too bulky.
- *Transposition:* by moving muscles out of their field of action into another area this improves the movement in another direction of gaze (Figures 12.9 and 12. 10). This is commonly used in VI nerve palsies where the superior and inferior rectus muscles are moved laterally to provide some abduction. The inferior oblique can be transposed anteriorly in order to transform its action from elevation into passive restriction of upgaze (Figure 13.3).

Sutures

The development of modern suture materials has led to an improvement in the outcome of squint surgery, with fewer complications associated with finer, more inert sutures. In standard squint surgery the extra-ocular muscles should be sutured with absorbable sutures (plain 6/0 polyglycolic acid sutures being the preferred option). In adjustable sutures surgery the optimum sutures are dyed 6/0 polyglycolic acid, as this material tends to run more smoothly through the tissues at the time of adjustment.

The conjunctiva should be closed with buried 8/0 polyglycolic acid.

Anaesthetic options for squint surgery

General anaesthesia

Principles: strabismus surgery is usually performed under general anaesthesia. Compared with other forms of eye surgery it may provoke a degree of nausea and vomiting postoperatively. One of the aims of anaesthesia should be to keep postoperative nausea to a minimum.

Anaesthetic regimen

- Preoperative medication is unnecessary in all cases except the most nervous adults and even then should be avoided in those undergoing adjustable suture surgery, if this is to take place on the same day.
- Ventilation via a laryngeal mask.
- Peroperative systemic short-acting opioid such as fentanyl.
- Peroperative systemic antiemetic.
- Peroperative non-steroidal anti-inflammatory drug (e.g. per rectum diclofenac).
- Use of systemic antimuscarinic if there is a bradycardia peroperatively, due to pulling on a muscle.

Surgical regimen to reduce surgical pain

- Confine conjunctival incisions, as far as possible, to the fornices and areas not in the interpalpebral fissure.
- Conjunctival sutures should be 8/0, absorbable and buried so that the ends lie subconjunctivally.
- Avoid damaging the corneal epithelium – this most often happens when suturing across the cornea, if the needle holders are allowed to lie too low or due to the traction sutures rubbing on the cornea.
- Subconjunctival infiltration of local anaesthetic over the surgically treated muscles is useful at the end of surgery in reducing the postoperative pain. Bupivicaine, a long-acting local anaesthetic agent, is ideal for this (0.1 ml).

Local anaesthesia

Indications

- Where there is a high anaesthetic risk but surgery is still desirable; e.g. intractable diplopia in an elderly patient.
- Patient request – some patients do not wish to have a general anaesthetic.

Topical anaesthetic

The entire squint operation can be performed under topical anaesthetic drops (e.g. proxymetacaine, benoxinate). This is usually used for the recession of one muscle and is well tolerated.

PROCEDURE

1. Instill topical anaesthetic drops (e.g. proxymetacaine, benoxinate) into the conjunctival sac.
2. Place a cotton bud soaked in anaesthetic agent over the area of conjunctival incision prior to commencing surgery.
3. There must be limited pulling on the muscle as sudden jerks cause severe discomfort.

This has the advantage of allowing adjustable sutures, if being performed, to be carried out as a 'one step' approach (see Chapter 14).

Local infiltration

PROCEDURE

1. Instill topical anaesthetic drops (e.g. benoxinate, proxymetacaine) into the conjunctival sac at the start of surgery.
2. Commence the conjunctival incision and through this infiltrate local anaesthetic (e.g. lidocaine with adrenaline) into the sub-Tenon's space, using a blunt cannula.
3. Continue with the strabismus surgery as planned.
4. Repeat step 2 during the operation if necessary.

Further reading

Apt L, Isenberg S, Gaffney EL. The oculocardiac reflex in strabismus surgery. *Am J Ophthalmol* 1973; **76**: 533–6

Helveston EM. The value of strabismus surgery. *Ophthal Surg* 1990; **21**: 311

Kim S, Yang Y, Kim J. Tolerance of patients and post-operative results; topical anaesthesia for strabismus surgery. *J Paediatr Ophthalmol Strabismus* 2000; **37**: 344–8

Mendel HG, Guarnieri KM, Sundt LM et al. The effects of ketorolac and fentanyl on post-operative vomiting and analgesic requirements in children undergoing strabismus surgery. *Anesth Analg* 1995; **80**: 1129

Rosenbaum AL, Santiago AP. *Clinical strabismus management – principles and surgical techniques*. WB Saunders & Co, Philadelphia. 1999

Splinter W, Noel LP, Roberts D *et al*. Antiemetic prophylaxis for strabismus surgery. *Can J Ophthalmol* 1994; **29**: 224

Tramer M, Moore A, McQuay H. Prevention of vomiting after paediatric strabismus surgery: a systematic review using the numbers needed to treat method. *Br J Anaesth* 1995; **75**: 556

Watcha MF, White PF. Post-operative nausea and vomiting: its etiology, treatment and prevention. *Anesthesiology* 1992; **77**: 162

Willshaw HE. Rectus muscle surgery – how to do it. *Trans Ophthalmol Soc UK* 1986; **105**: 583–8

4

Surgical anatomy

This chapter looks at the anatomy of the extraocular muscles with particular emphasis on aspects which are of relevance to planning and executing surgical treatment of strabismus.

Anatomy of the extraocular muscles

Actions of the extraocular muscles

Anatomy of the extraocular muscles

Origins

All the muscles take their origin from the back of the orbit, except the inferior oblique, which arises from a tubercle on the anterior inferior orbital wall, just lateral to the lacrimal fossa (Figure 4.1). This lies

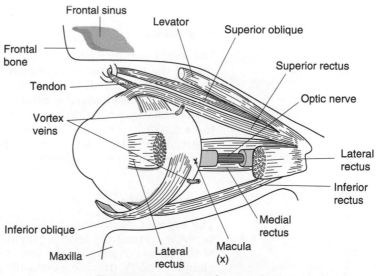

Figure 4.1 Extraocular muscles

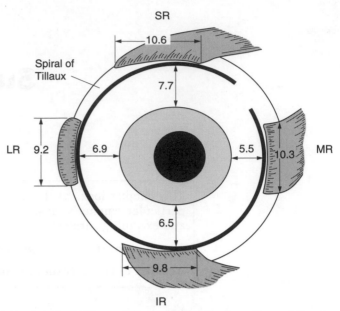

Figure 4.2 Spiral of Tillaux. The widths of the insertions of the four rectus muscles and the distance of these from the limbus (in mm)

directly beneath the trochlea, which is the effective origin of the superior oblique, since its tendon runs through this pulley system. The four recti change direction slightly at about the equator of the globe, by means of attachments to the orbital fascia. This alters their line of action slightly and explains why transposition procedures are not quite as effective as one might expect.

Insertions

The recti insert by means of tendons that are roughly 10 mm in width – that of the lateral rectus is slightly thinner, at about 9 mm. The insertions vary in their distance from the limbus with the superior rectus lying the furthest back (the spiral of Tillaux – Figure 4.2). The insertions of the obliques are behind the equator. They vary from 7 mm in width to as much as 18 mm. The superior oblique has more variation in its insertion than the inferior, which probably accounts for the frequency of congenital superior oblique 'palsy'.

Nerve supply

The superior division of the III (oculomotor) cranial nerve supplies the superior rectus (and levator palpabrae superioris); the inferior division of the III nerve supplies the inferior rectus, medial rectus and inferior oblique. The IV (trochlear) cranial nerve supplies the superior oblique. The VI (abducens) cranial nerve supplies the lateral rectus.

Blood supply

All the extraocular muscles take their blood supply from the ophthalmic artery. The blood supply of the recti, in addition, supplies the anterior segment via the anterior ciliary arteries. The lateral rectus has only one of these arteries, lying in the lower part of its insertion – the other three recti have two, lying at the margins of the insertions. Fluorescein angiography has demonstrated that most of the blood to the anterior segment comes from the anterior ciliary arteries of the vertical recti. Surgery to more than two rectus muscles can lead to anterior segment ischaemia.

Important relations

- The superior rectus shares a common tendon of origin with the levator palpebrae superioris (Figure 4.1).
- The lateral rectus has fascial attachments to the inferior oblique muscle which is inserted along its lower border.
- The inferior oblique has fascial attachments to the inferior rectus as it passes under this muscle (Figure 4.1).
- The inferior rectus has attachments to the lower lid retractors, so large recessions of this muscle are usually accompanied by retraction of the lower lid.
- The medial rectus has no fascial attachments to other muscles and can therefore retract to the orbital apex if severed from the globe.
- The superior oblique passes through the trochlea, which lies on the frontal bone adjacent to the frontal sinus, disease of which can affect the function of the superior oblique (Figure 4.1).
- The insertions of the two obliques, lying so posterior, are adjacent to the emissary vortex veins, which must be identified and preserved during any surgery (Figure 4.1).

Common anomalies of the extraocular muscles

- Diffuse insertion of a rectus muscle may make hooking of the muscle difficult and cause an unexpected surgical result.
- Partially bifid belly of a rectus muscle may allow the strabismus hook to pass through a division rather than the entire muscle.
- Absence of an extraocular muscle is rare, but well described, particularly of the superior rectus and superior oblique muscles.
- The fibres of the superior oblique tendon can appear very diaphanous, so that the inexperienced surgeon might be forgiven for thinking that this muscle is absent, but a careful search usually reveals the tendon.
- Abnormal insertion of the medial and lateral rectus muscles (either congenital or surgically induced) may produce an A or V pattern.
- If either of the horizontal rectus muscles is very tight, it may interfere with vertical movements of the globe, or produce vertical

movements by slipping over the globe as it rotates (so-called 'leash effect').

Ligaments

The extraocular muscles are enveloped in a sheath over their entire length, but which becomes distinct only anteriorly. The sheath of the inferior rectus is attached to the sheath of the inferior oblique where they cross. The sheaths of the obliques are attached to the globe by fine fibrous connections, so that there is not complete loss of function of these muscles after free tenotomies. The rectus muscles have expansions of their sheaths at the point at which they turn towards the globe at the equator. These are the check ligaments and the outer, orbital, fibres of the recti insert into them – the inner, global, fibres insert into the sclera. They should be dissected from the muscle during surgery.

Actions of the extraocular muscles

The extraocular muscles act together in order to produce smooth eye movements over a wide range. The relative contributions of each muscle to the various ocular positions need to be understood (Figure 4.3). The vertical rectus muscles and obliques have complex actions which vary depending on the horizontal position of the eyes (Figures 4.4 and 4.5). The horizontal recti have only one primary action.

Medial rectus

- Adducts the eye (Figure 4.6)

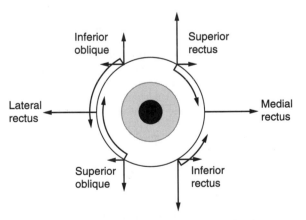

Figure 4.3 The actions of the extraocular muscles: the length of the arrows shows their relative strengths

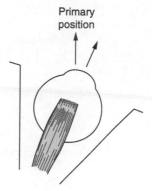

Figure 4.4   In abduction the vertical recti have a vertical action only

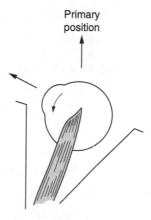

Figure 4.5   In adduction the vertical recti become tortors of the eye

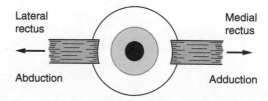

Figure 4.6   Action of the lateral and medial rectus muscles

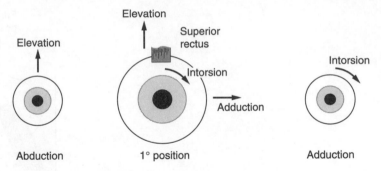

Figure 4.7 Superior rectus action

Lateral rectus

- Abducts the eye (Figure 4.6)

Superior rectus

The superior rectus has three actions (Figure 4.7):

- elevation
- intorsion
- adduction.

The relative strengths of these actions depend upon the direction of gaze – in extreme adduction the intorting power of the superior rectus is enhanced and in abduction its power of intorsion is lost and it becomes an elevator.

Inferior rectus

The inferior rectus has three actions (Figure 4.8):

- depression
- extorsion
- adduction.

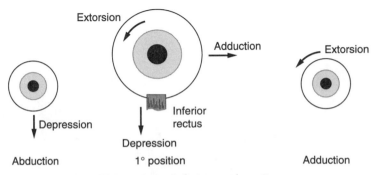

Figure 4.8 Inferior rectus action

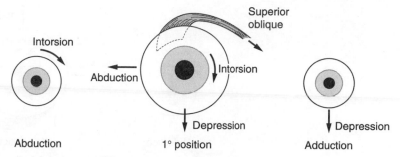

Figure 4.9   Superior oblique action

The inferior rectus is most efficient at extorsion when the eye is in adduction; when the eye is in a position of abduction the muscle becomes a pure depressor.

Superior oblique

The superior oblique has three actions (Figure 4.9):

- intorsion
- depression
- abduction.

The superior oblique is the principal intortor of the eye; this action is produced by the anterior fibres of the tendon (Figure 4.10). Its most posterior fibres mediate depression. In extreme adduction it becomes a pure depressor – in abduction it is a pure intortor.

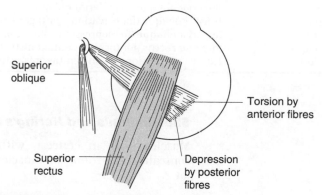

Figure 4.10   Actions of different aspects of the superior oblique

Inferior oblique

The inferior oblique has three actions (Figure 4.11):

- extorsion
- elevation
- abduction.

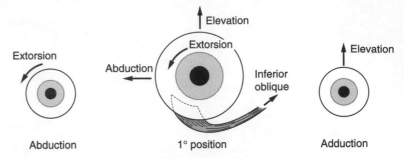

Figure 4.11 Inferior oblique action

The inferior oblique is the principal extortor of the eye, with secondary effects of elevation in adduction. In extreme adduction it becomes a pure elevator – in abduction a pure extortor.

Ipsilateral synergists

Table 4.1 lists the muscles in the same eye which share a similar action.

Table 4.1 Ipsilateral synergists: these are the muscles in the same eye which share a similar action

Muscle	Ipsilateral synergists	Action
Medial rectus	Superior rectus and inferior rectus	Adduction
Lateral rectus	Superior oblique and inferior oblique	Abduction
Superior rectus	Inferior oblique (for elevation – antagonistic for torsion)	Elevation
Inferior rectus	Superior oblique (for depression – antagonistic for torsion)	Depression
Superior oblique	Superior rectus (for torsion – antagonistic for depression)	Incyclotorsion
Inferior oblique	Inferior rectus (for torsion – antagonistic for elevation)	Excycotorsion

Sherrington's and Hering's laws

Muscles work in concert, with cooperation between ipsilateral and contralateral groups of muscles, abiding Sherrington's and Hering's laws.

Sherrington's law of reciprocal innervation

Contraction of a muscle is accompanied by relaxation of its ipsilateral antagonist muscle. Thus relaxation of the lateral rectus occurs simultaneously with contraction of the medial rectus (and similarly for other ipsilateral antagonists), ensuring smooth movements of the eyes.

Ipsilateral antagonists

These are the muscles in the same eye that have opposing actions and which obey Sherrington's law:

Medial rectus (adductor)	Lateral rectus (abductor)
Superior rectus (elevator in abduction)	Inferior rectus (depressor in abduction)
Superior oblique (intortor)	Inferior oblique (extortor)
Superior oblique (depressor in adduction)	Inferior oblique (elevator in adduction)

Hering's law of equal innervation

In binocular movements, equal contractions occur in the muscles that are contralateral synergists. If both muscles are normal, equal movements of the two eyes occur. If one muscle is weak, the extra drive to make this muscle contract also drives its synergist muscle in the other eye that therefore tends to overact.

Contralateral synergists

This term refers to the pair of muscles, one from each eye, that has the same field of action, obeying Hering's Law:

Medial rectus (adduction)	Lateral rectus (abduction)
Inferior rectus (depression in abduction)	Superior oblique (depression in adduction)
Superior rectus (elevation in abduction)	Inferior oblique (elevation in adduction)
Superior oblique and superior rectus (incyclotorsion)	Inferior oblique and inferior rectus (excyclotorsion)

Further reading

Apt L. An anatomical evaluation of rectus muscle insertions. *Trans Am Ophthalmol Soc* 1980; **78**: 365

Boeder P. Co-operative action of the extraocular muscles. *Br J Ophthalmol* 1962; **46**: 397

Duke-Elder S, Wybar KC. The anatomy of the visual system. *System of ophthalmology*, Vol 2, Mosby-Year Book, Inc, St Louis. 1961

Gordon OE. A study of primary and auxiliary ocular rotations. *Trans Exp Ophthalmol* 1988; **58**: 553

Leigh RJ, Zee DS. *The neurology of eye movements*, 2nd edn. FA Davis Company, Philadelphia. 1992

Scobee RC. Anatomic factors in the etiology of strabismus. *Am J Ophthalmol* 1948; **31**: 781

Sevel P. The origins and insertions of the extraocular muscles: development, histologic features and clinical significance. *Trans Am Ophthalmol Soc* 1986; **84**: 488

PART 2
What to do

5

Concomitant eso-deviations

Concomitant eso-deviations are classified as follows:

Primary esotropia
- Intermittent
  - accommodative
    - fully accommodative
    - convergence excess esotropia
  - non-accommodative
    - near esotropia
    - esophoria – decompensating
    - cyclical esotropia
- Constant
  - accommodative
    - partially accommodative
  - non-acccommodative
    - early onset esotropia (infantile or congenital esotropia)
    - nystagmus block esotropia
    - sudden onset esotropia (late onset esotropia)
    - micro-csotropia

Secondary esotropia: due to poor vision in the convergent eye

Consecutive esotropia: following previous exotropia (either with or without surgery)
- immediate postoperative
- non-specific

Primary esotropia

Primary concomitant esotropias commonly have an intermittent onset. These are usually divided into those that have an accommodative element and those that are non-accommodative.

Intermittent accommodative esotropia

The convergent strabismus is secondary to a high accommodative drive due to:

- uncorrected hypermetropia (fully accommodative esotropia, which is a refractive aetiology)
- high AC/A ratio (convergence excess esotropia, which is a non-refractive aetiology).

Separating refractive and non-refractive accommodative esotropia can be difficult, as there is commonly overlap between the two conditions, giving a mixed picture, due to the presence of hypermetropia and a high AC/A ratio.

Fully accommodative esotropia (refractive)

CLINICAL FEATURES

- Esotropia, which becomes apparent when accommodation is exerted (usually intermittent at first, becoming more obvious when the patient is tired or unwell; it may become constant if not treated).
- Age of onset 1–4 years.
- Onset may be precipitated by illness or trauma.
- Hypermetropia of any amount.
- No residual esotropia for near or distance when wearing full hypermetropic spectacle correction.
- Normal binocular function when squint not present, although may develop a microtropia (see below), or may become constant if left untreated.
- Amblyopia rare (may occur due to anisometropia or if the squint becomes constant).
- Familial tendency.

DIFFERENTIAL DIAGNOSIS

- Convergence excess esotropia
- Near esotropia
- Decompensating esophoria

MANAGEMENT (FIGURE 5.1)

Non-surgical treatment   The treatment of this condition is non-surgical.

1. Cycloplegic refraction, with prescription of *full* hypermetropic correction, subtracting only the working distance (see Chapter 2).
2. Surgery should *not* be performed, despite parental requests, unless there is decompensation to a constant strabismus with *maximum* spectacle correction in place.
3. Orthoptic treatment may be helpful in teaching control of the deviation without spectacle correction in older children – so that they can control the deviation without glasses.

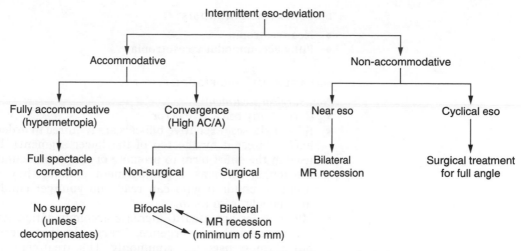

Figure 5.1 Management of intermittent eso-deviations

Surgical treatment: (for decompensated fully accommodative esotropia only) Occasionally fully accommodative squints do break down after a period of control. Ensure the full refractive correction is in place and increase this if possible (atropine refraction may be required). However, under these circumstances it may not be possible to regain control without surgical correction and this should be carried out as soon as possible in order to retain binocular function.

- Bilateral medial rectus recessions, aiming to fully correct the near angle of deviation (Figure 5.1, see also Chapter 12)
- Undercorrection is common so err on the generous side.

The aim of surgery is to correct the angle *with glasses on* (unless a low hypermetrope, then can aim to get out of glasses completely) for a functional result.

Convergence excess esotropia (high AC/A ratio)

This is an intermittent esotropia that occurs secondary to a high AC/A ratio.

CLINICAL FEATURES

- Esotropia in which the angle of deviation is larger for near to an accommodative target than it is for distance, by at least 10 dioptres.
- Usually manifest for near and small latent angle for distance.
- Age of onset 1–4 years.
- Binocular function present for distance and when corrected for near, although may develop a microtropia.
- High AC/A ratio (higher than normal range of 3.5–5.1).
- Amblyopia rare.
- Minimal hypermetropia, although there may be an element of anisometropia.

DIFFERENTIAL DIAGNOSIS
- Near esotropia
- Fully accommodative esotropia

MANAGEMENT (SEE FIGURE 5.1)

Non-surgical treatment
- Correct any refractive error
- Bifocal glasses (executive bifocals are required in order that the visual axis is bisected by the top of the lower segment). Bifocals may be used in the short term to promote or retain binocular function or in the longer term as a management option. They are really only useful in children who can read and younger children tend to get little benefit from them.
- Miotic drops are used to increase accommodation without inducing accommodative convergence. Previously they were very popular, but are now used less commonly. This treatment is rarely a long-term solution (see Chapter 2).

Surgical treatment
- Bilateral medial rectus recessions of at least 5 mm (for all angles of strabismus up to 35 dioptres) (Table 5.1(e), see also Chapter 12).
- For squints >35 dioptres, do 1 mm more for each 5 dioptres greater than this to a maximum of 12.5 mm from limbus.

Despite apparently adequate amounts of surgery, some patients remain convergent for near. Options in such cases include:

- Bifocal glasses – with the aim gradually to wean them out of these over the next few months
- Botulinum toxin injection to each medial rectus

Table 5.1 Esotropia – a guide to surgical treatment. Each patient requires an individual surgical approach to the management of their squint, but the following measurements may be of assistance *as a guide*, particularly for those beginning strabismus surgery

Angle of squint	Bilateral MR recessions	or	MR recession/LR resection	
20 D	3.5 mm		4 mm	5 mm
30 D	4.5 mm		5 mm	6 mm
40 D	5 mm		5 mm	7.5 mm
50 D	6 mm		5.5 mm	8 mm

a) These measurements are only for concomitant deviations, with no underlying muscle or neurological pathology or previous surgery
b) The measurements for recessions are taken from the insertion of the muscle
c) The measurements should be altered based on the surgeon's personal results
d) If the horizonatal angle is greater for near than distance relatively more should be done to the medial rectus than the lateral rectus, and vice versa
e) If the AC/C ratio is high (>5:1) in a child with an accommodative esotropia, bilateral medial recessions of at lease 5 mm should be undertaken, even for small deviations
f) Aim to slightly undercorrect secondary estropia, or those with poor binocular function
g) For angles >50 dioptres perform surgery to more than 2 horizontal recti

- Re-recession of each medial rectus to a maximum of 12.5–13 mm from limbus (although this may result in consecutive divergence in the long term)
- Faden operation to each medial rectus
- Medial tenotomy of each medial rectus.

The aim of surgery is a functional result for near and distance.

Intermittent non-accommodative esotropia

Near esotropia

This is a concomitant eso-deviation which is manifest for near, but straight or latent for distance and resembles a convergence excess esotropia, except that the AC/A ratio is normal. This is thought to be due to increased tone in baseline convergence.

CLINICAL FEATURES

- Onset 2–5 years.
- Esotropia which is manifest for near and a small latent angle for distance.
- Angle for near usually moderate to large.
- Normal motor and sensory fusion for distance.
- Normal AC/A ratio.
- Amblyopia rare.
- Rarely significant refractive error.

DIFFERENTIAL DIAGNOSIS

- Convergence excess esotropia (differentiated from this by the presence of a normal AC/A ratio.

MANAGEMENT (SEE FIGURE 5.1)

Non-surgical treatment   Correction of any refractive error.

Surgical treatment   The treatment is surgical, as unlike convergence excess esotropia bifocals and miotics are unhelpful.

- Bilateral medial rectus recessions, aiming to correct the angle for near (see Table 5.1, see also Chapter 12)

The aim of surgery is a functional result.

Esophoria (decompensating)

Esophoria is a latent convergent squint. Binocular single vision is achieved by adequate negative fusional vergence (the motor ability to diverge). Esophoria is asymptomatic in the majority of people, but may decompensate and become symptomatic.

Decompensation usually occurs spontaneously, but may be precipitated by a change in refractive status or spectacle correction, by excessive visual demands or by ill health.

CLINICAL FEATURES

- Gradual, vague onset of symptoms (unless onset due to a sudden precipitant, e.g. change of glasses, head injury).
- Age of onset anytime – children or adults.
- Symptoms may be variable, e.g. eye strain, headache, blurring of vision, intermittent diplopia, closure of one eye for visually demanding activities.
- Equal vision.
- Cover test reveals reduced rate of recovery of esophoria (recovery absent in fully decompensated cases).
- BVA reduced.
- Reduced or absent negative motor fusion range (the ability to overcome base in prisms).
- Evidence of sensory fusion.
- Angle of deviation usually larger for near or distance
  - larger for near (near esophoria, with symptoms for close work)
  - larger for distance (distance esophoria, with symptoms for distance activities)
  - occasionally the angle may be equal for near and distance (non-specific esophoria).
- Symptoms tend to occur with increased visual demand for the angle of maximal deviation.

DIFFERENTIAL DIAGNOSIS

- Fully accommodative esotropia
- Convergence excess esotropia
- Decompensating micro-esotropia

MANAGEMENT

Non-surgical treatment Treatment is offered if the decompensating/decompensated esophoria produces symptoms.

- Refraction – full hypermetropic correction prescribed, ensure that current spectacles are correct.
- Orthoptic treatment – exercises to improve the negative fusional amplitude.
- Base out prisms – not recommended as a long-term solution as the requirement for prisms tends to increase gradually with the passage of time, but can be useful in elderly or unwell patients. Always use the smallest size of prism that relieves symptoms.
- Botulinum toxin – injection of the medial rectus muscle can be effective in reducing the angle of deviation and restoring binocular single vision; this, in turn, stimulates improvement in the motor fusion range and results in fewer symptoms and better control of the esophoria. This result is frequently long-standing, with beneficial

effects long after the pharmacological effects of the toxin have worn off, and may result in a cure of the condition.

Surgical treatment   Surgery is recommended for patients who remain symptomatic despite appropriate conservative treatment. This is more likely to be required in those with large angled deviations, those with near esophorias associated with a high AC/A ratio and esophorias that are larger in the distance. In children surgery is recommended if there is evidence that binocular function is being compromised by the esophoria.

Surgery should be carried out using adjustable sutures where possible (see Chapter 14) and consists of:

- Unilateral medial rectus recession – for small near esophorias (<15 dioptres) (see Chapter 12)
- Bilateral medial rectus recessions – for moderate to large near esophorias (see Chapter 12)
- Unilateral medial rectus recession and lateral rectus resection – for distance or non-specific esophorias (see Chapter 12).

The amount of surgery performed is based on the maximum angle of the deviation (see Table 5.1). The aim of surgery is to correct the deviation fully.

Cyclical esotropia

This is an eso-deviation which is intermittent in time, in that it is manifest for some periods of time and absent for others on a cyclical basis.

CLINICAL FEATURES

- Onset 3–6 years.
- Manifest deviation usually for 24 hours followed by 24 hours of no deviation (period of the cycle may vary, but is constant for each individual).
- Angle usually equal for distance and near.
- Binocular single vision present when not manifest.
- Suppression present when manifest.
- No significant refractive error.
- Amblyopia rare.
- Commonly progresses to become a constantly manifest deviation.

DIFFERENTIAL DIAGNOSIS

- The diagnosis is usually not in doubt, but the clinical features may be simulated by intermittent control of an accommodative esotropia or decompensating esophoria, although a clear history should distinguish these.

MANAGEMENT

Non-surgical treatment

- Full cycloplegic refraction

Surgical treatment This is the treatment of choice and should be performed prior to constant breakdown in the deviation.

- A unilateral medial rectus recession combined with a lateral rectus resection (see Chapter 12).
- The amount of surgery performed aims to correct the maximum size of the deviation when manifest (see Table 5.1).

The aim of surgery is to correct fully the size of the manifest deviation to regain normal binocular single vision.

Constant accommodative esotropia

Partially accommodative esotropia

This may be an entity in its own right, or secondary to a long-standing untreated or undercorrected fully accommodative esotropia which has developed amblyopia and loss of binocular function.

CLINICAL FEATURES

- Age of onset 2–5 years. Constant unilateral esotropia, with residual esotropia with full hypermetropic correction in place.
- Poor/no binocular function for near or distance, with suppression of the squinting eye.
- Amblyopia of the esotropic eye.
- Hypermetropia, which may be asymmetrical.
- Familial tendency.

DIFFERENTIAL DIAGNOSIS

- Undercorrected fully accommodative esotropia

MANAGEMENT

Non-surgical treatment
- Full cycloplegic refraction with prescription of glasses
- Treatment of amblyopia

Surgical treatment Surgery principally for cosmesis, although it may promote some degree of abnormal binocular function, especially in younger children. Spectacle wear and amblyopia treatment may need to continue following surgery.

- Surgery is usually directed to the amblyopic eye.
- Medial rectus recession with a lateral rectus resection aiming to undercorrect slightly the deviation (see Table 5.1 and Chapter 12).

- If there is a large difference between the angle of squint for distance viewing compared to near, the surgery can be tailored to allow for this, e.g. more medial rectus recession is performed if the near angle is greater and less lateral rectus resection.
- Aim to correct the angle with glasses on if significant hypermetropia or astigmatism – aim to get out of glasses if <3 dioptres or low degree of astigmatism that is not affecting vision.

The aim of surgery is an improvement in cosmesis. In some cases correcting the angle may provide an opportunity for the development of some gross abnormal binocular function, especially in the younger children who are still visually immature. Such a result is not guaranteed, but if this develops it may promote a more stable result in the long term.

Constant non-accommodative esotropia

Early-onset esotropia (also known as congenital or infantile esotropia)

This is an esotropia which is present from early in life with specific clinical characteristics. The underlying aetiology is unclear, but is probably a neurodevelopmental anomaly affecting the oculomotor and visual sensory systems. Other areas of brain development are normal.

CLINICAL FEATURES

- Early onset of squint (before 6 months of age).
- Large angle esotropia for near and distance (usually 40 dioptres or more).
- No binocular function.
- Concomitant, but may develop habitual reduction in abduction due to 'tripartite' or 'cross' fixation.
- Amblyopia uncommon as the eyes usually freely alternate (but may develop amblyopia after surgical correction and therefore require careful observation).
- Significant refractive error uncommon.
- Asymmetric OKN responses (i.e. the infantile responses are preserved).
- Inferior oblique overaction may be present, but usually develops months/years after onset.
- DVD may be present, but may develop months/years after onset.
- Latent nystagmus may be present.

DIFFERENTIAL DIAGNOSIS

- Congenital VI nerve palsy
- Duane's retraction syndrome
- Nystagmus block esotropia
- Secondary squint due to poor vision in one eye

MANAGEMENT

Non-surgical treatment
- Treatment is usually surgical although any hypermetropia (>2.0 dioptres), or significant anisometropia (>1.0 dioptres) should be treated with glasses first to optimize visual acuity.
- Amblyopia is rare, but if present (identified by lack of free alternation or grating activities) should be treated prior to surgery, with very careful supervision due to the young age of the child.

Surgical treatment   Surgery is the usual form of treatment.
There is no consensus of opinion as to the best timing for surgery – 'early' (9–18 months of age) or 'late' (usually before starting school at around 4 years of age) – either option is acceptable, as each has advantages and disadvantages. Very early surgery for this condition (<6 months) remains controversial.

- Bilateral recessions of the medial recti are the preferred operation (commonly to 11.5 mm from limbus – this is approximately equivalent to a 6 mm recession from the muscle insertion, but is taken from the limbus in children as it is more accurate). Measurements aim to correct the full angle and this will treat up to 45–50 dioptres (see Table 5.1 and Chapter 12).
- Recession of the conjunctiva will augment the surgical correction, if the angle is large (>45 dioptres).
- If the angle is very large (>50 dioptres), a 5–7 mm resection of one lateral rectus should be added, but the medial rectus recessions should be reduced to 10.5 mm from limbus – equivalent to 5 mm recessions.
- Horizontal rectus muscle surgery may need to be combined with surgery to weaken the inferior oblique or to treat DVD. This may take place simultaneously or at a later date.

The aim of surgery is to correct within 10 dioptres of straight, but the direction of the final outcome depends on the timing of surgery:

- In early surgery (9–18 months), the ideal immediate postoperative result is a slight divergence, as it is hoped that this may stimulate the suppressed retina and promote some degree of binocular function
- In late surgery (4 years or older), there is a risk of the development of consecutive exotropia – a slight residual esotropia is preferable.

Amblyopia may develop following surgery and therefore careful follow-up is essential, with appropriate treatment if required.

Nystagmus block esotropia

This esotropia develops in patients with congenital nystagmus in order to enhance monocular acuity by damping the nystagmus using convergence.

CLINICAL FEATURES

- Presents in early life (<6 months).
- Variable angle esotropia, which becomes larger on fixating an object (for near or distance).
- Abnormal head posture because of tendency to use either eye in adduction only, even when monocular and using a face turn away from object of regard.
- Nystagmus develops on abduction of either eye, which damps on adduction.
- Concomitant, but patient reluctant to abduct due to increasing nystagmus in that position.
- Significant refractive error rare.
- Amblyopia may occur as a preference for fixation with one eye often develops.
- Pupils often small.

DIFFERENTIAL DIAGNOSIS

- Early onset esotropia
- Congenital VI nerve palsy
- Duane's retraction syndrome
- Early-onset accommodative esotropia

MANAGEMENT

Non-surgical treatment

- Treat significant refractive error, if present
- Treat amblyopia

Surgical treatment   Treatment of the strabismus is surgical.
- Bilateral medial rectus recessions (usually to 11.5 or 12 mm from limbus) (see Chapter 12)
- Surgery may be ineffective and re-operation in the form of Faden suture to both medial recti may be required

The aim of surgery is to reduce the esotropia by allowing dampening of the nystagmus with less convergence. A functional result with binocular vision is unlikely.

Sudden onset esotropia (late onset esotropia)

This is an esotropia which develops suddenly in an older child (usually >4 years old) with diplopia. There may be a past history of previous squint or recent occlusion of one eye (due to injury or inflammation).

CLINICAL FEATURES

- Age of onset 4–12 years.
- Sudden onset (may be spontaneous or following a minor incident such as a small bump on the head).

- Diplopia present, with normal vision in both eyes.
- Evidence of binocular potential when angle corrected.
- Relatively large angle of deviation – near and distance.
- Full range of movements of both eyes – no incomitance.
- There may be a family history of other types of esotropia.
- Significant refractive error rare.

The sudden onset of a squint in an older child is concerning and the presence of any of the following features should raise suspicion and suggest that further neurological examination, investigation and imaging are required:

- Any signs of incomitance
- Any form of nystagmus
- Lack of any evidence of any binocular function
- Suggestion of poor divergence (distance angle measures more than the near angle)
- Presence of an A or V pattern
- Any other neurological signs or symptoms.

DIFFERENTIAL DIAGNOSIS

- Decompensated microtropia
- Decompensated esophoria
- Decompensated unrecognized accommodative esotropia

MANAGEMENT

Initial management Examination and investigation:

- Refract and carry out full orthoptic assessment including motor fusional ranges and sensory binocular function
- Full ophthalmic examination
- Full neurological examination
- Neuroimaging if indicated.

Non-surgical treatment
- Uni- or bilateral injection of botulinum toxin to the medial rectus muscles should be carried out as soon as possible. This usually permanently corrects the squint as the restoration of single binocular vision enables the patient to continue aligning the eyes even after the botulinum toxin has worn off.

Surgical treatment If botulinum toxin is unavailable or if the squint recurs after an injection of toxin, surgery should be carried out:

- A medial rectus recession, combined with a lateral rectus resection, aiming to correct the full angle of squint (see Chapter 12).

The aim of treatment is a functional result, with restoration of binocular single vision.

Micro-esotropia

Micro-esotropia is a small-angled squint, with evidence of binocular function, although this is reduced in quantity and quality. This may decompensate and require surgical treatment or micro-esotropia may be the result of surgical treatment for accommodative esotropia.

CLINICAL FEATURES

- Small-angled esotropia (<10 dioptres).
- Anisometropia common.
- Mild amblyopia in the affected eye, although denser amblyopia may occur.
- Eccentric para-foveal fixation in the amblyopic eye.
- Abnormal binocular vision with reduced motor range and sensory function.
- May be an isolated entity or associated with accommodative esotropia.
- Positive 4 dioptre prism test.

MANAGEMENT

Non-surgical treatment
- Correction of refractive error
- Treatment of amblyopia
- Orthoptic treatment may help to strengthen control

Surgical treatment Surgery is only indicated for a microtropia if it decompensates to become a manifest strabismus. It should be carried out soon after the decompensation takes place.

- Surgery is usually carried out on the amblyopic eye
- A medial rectus recession combined with a lateral rectus resection to correct the full angle of deviation (see Table 5.1 and Chapter 12)

The aim of surgery is to attempt to restore some degree of binocular function.

Secondary esotropia

An esotropia caused by poor vision in the squinting eye. In children secondary squints are commonly esotropic (in adults they are more commonly exotropic).

CLINICAL FEATURES

- An esotropia of any size of angle.
- Poor vision in the esotropic eye.
- Full range of movements of both eyes.

- Esotropia with an amblyopic eye

MANAGEMENT

Non-surgical treatment   Full ophthalmic examination to identify the cause of visual loss. Treatment of the visual loss if this is possible (e.g. cataract extraction).

- If vision can be restored, the treatment of choice is an injection of botulinum toxin to the medial rectus of the esotropic eye. This is successful in restoring a functional result in a significant proportion of patients.

Surgical treatment   Surgery is the management of choice in those with persistent reduction in vision:

- Medial rectus recession and lateral rectus resection to the eye with poor vision (see Chapter 12)
- Leave slightly esotropic as will tend to diverge.

The aim of surgery is a long-term cosmetic result.

Consecutive esotropia

This is an esotropia that occurs in a patient with a previous history of exotropia or exophoria. This tends to occur under two sets of circumstances:

1. Immediate postoperative – *occurring immediately* following surgery for exotropia (commonly intermittent distance exotropia), where the surgical aim is a small overcorrection, but the result is slightly more than desired
2. Non-specific – occurring either spontaneously, or many months or years after surgery for exotropia. This is less common and is more likely to occur if patients with an exo-deviation develop myopia which requires correction, usually in adolescence or early adult life.

Immediate postoperative consecutive esotropia

CLINICAL FEATURES
- Recent surgery for previous exo-deviation.
- Esotropia often small, but may vary in size.
- Full range of movements.
- Patient may be quite distressed by troublesome diplopia.

DIFFERENTIAL DIAGNOSIS

The diagnosis is usually not in doubt, but needs to be differentiated from a slipped or lost muscle (see Chapter 16).

MANAGEMENT

Non-surgical treatment

- In the immediate postoperative period the patient should be patched for symptomatic relief (alternate eyes daily) and observed as the deviation is likely to improve spontaneously within 2 weeks of the surgery
- If it persists >2 weeks then the recovery period may be prolonged and treatment in the form of either
  - prisms to neutralize the angle, with the plan gradually to reduce the power over the next few months as the angle spontaneously reduces
  - bifocal spectacles, to reduce the angle for near
  - botulinum toxin treatment to one medial rectus muscle (see Chapter 15)
- Observe carefully for the development of amblyopia in children and treat if required.

Surgical treatment   In cases that persist >6–9 months (or earlier if toxin is not available) surgery is required.

- This usually involves re-advancing one of the recessed lateral rectus muscles, but each case is different and the procedure will depend on the pattern of deviation.

Non-specific secondary esotropia

CLINICAL FEATURES

- History of previous exo-deviation, either treated surgically or not.
- Esotropia of any size of angle.
- May be asymptomatic, or accompanied by diplopia.
- Accompanying A or V pattern common.
- Slight limitation of abduction common, especially in those who have previously undergone surgical correction of the initial exotropia.

DIFFERENTIAL DIAGNOSIS

- VI nerve palsy
- Decompensating microtropia
- Decompensating esophoria

MANAGEMENT

Non-surgical treatment   Ensure that refraction is accurate (any myopia is not overcorrected).

Surgical treatment   Surgical treatment involves recession of the medial rectus and resection (or re-advancement in previous surgical cases) of the lateral rectus of the squinting eye (see Chapter 12).

Further reading

Chamberlain W. Cyclic esotropia. *Am Orthoptic J* 1968; **18**: 31

Good WV, da Sa LCF, Lyons CJ, Hoyt CS. Monocular visual outcome in untreated early onset esotropia. *Br J Ophthalmol* 1993; **77**: 492–494

Hayati T, Kemal D, Abdullah O. Long-term results of bimedial rectus recessions in infantile esotropia. *J Pediatr Ophthalmol Strabismus* 1999; **36**: 201–5

Ing MR. Early surgical alignment for congenital esotropia. *Ophthalmology* 1983; **90**: 132–5

Keenan JM, Willshaw HE. Outcome of strabismus surgery in congenital esotropia. *Br J Ophthalmol* 1992; **76**: 342–5

Lang J. Normosensorial late convergent squint. In: Mein J, Moore S (eds). *Orthoptics, research & practice. Transactions of the Fourth International Orthoptic Congress, 1979, Berne*, Henry Kimpton, London. 1981; 230–3

Lymburn EG, MacEwen CJ. Botulinum toxin in the management of heterophoria. *Br Orthoptic J* 1994; **51**: 38

Parks MM, Wheeler MB. Concomitant esodeviations. In: Tasman W, Jaeger EA (eds). *Duane's clinical ophthalmology*, JB Lippincott. 1989; vol 1 ch 12

Raab EL. Hypermetropia in accommodative eso deviation. *J Pediatr Ophthalmol Strabismus* 1984; **21**: 64–8

Riordan-Eva P, Vickers SF, McCarry B, Lee JP. Cyclical strabismus without binocular function. *J Pediatr Ophthalmol Strabismus* 1993; **30**: 106–8

Roper-Hall MJ, Yapp JMS. Alternate day squint. In: *Transactions of the First International Congress of Orthoptics*, Kimpton, London. 1968; 262–71

Taylor DM. How early is early surgery in the management of strabismus. *Arch Ophthalmol* 1963; **70**: 752–6

Tolun H , Dikici V, Ozkiris A. Long-term results of bimedial rectus recessions in infantile esotropia. *J Pediatr Ophthalmol Strabismus* 1999; **36**: 201–5

von Noorden GK. The nystagmus compensation (blockage) syndrome. *Am J Ophthalmol* 1976; **82**: 283–90

von Noorden GK. A reassessment of infantile esotropia. XLIV Edward Jackson memorial lecture. *Am J Ophthalmol* 1988; **105**: 1–10

von Noorden GK, Jenkins RH. Non accommodative convergence excess. *Am J Ophthalmol* 1986; **100**: 70–3

6

Concomitant exo-deviations

Concomitant exo-deviations are classified as follows:

Primary exotropia
- Intermittent
  - distance
  - near
  - non-specific
- Exophoria (decompensating)
- Constant

Secondary exotropia – due to poor vision in the diverging eye

Consecutive exotropia – following previous esotropia (either with or without surgery)

Primary exotropia

Primary exo-deviations are commonly intermittent, although with time they may decompensate and become constant. They are classified depending on the distance at which the deviation is larger or manifest.

Intermittent exotropia (distance)

The cause of intermittent exotropia of the distance type is unknown, but may be supranuclear in origin. There may be associated anatomical features of the eyes, extraocular muscles and orbits which favour divergence (e.g. wide interpupillary distance).

CLINICAL FEATURES
- Intermittent exotropia for distance, exophoria for near (angle measures >10 prism dioptres for distance than it measures for near).
- Onset in early life (6–18 months).
- Good stereoacuity for near, but reduced motor fusion range for near.
- Dense suppression for distance, although may report panoramic vision.

- Concomitant, but may demonstrate lateral incomitance (angle of deviation decreases on lateral gaze).
- Tendency to close one eye in bright light.
- Usually asymptomatic (deviation noticed by others, especially when day dreaming, tired or unwell).
- Amblyopia rare.
- Refractive error rare.
- May deteriorate with time to become constantly manifest.

There are two main types of distance exotropia:

1. True divergence excess – the near angle is smaller than the distance angle (normal AC/A ratio)
2. Simulated divergence excess – the underlying angle is the same for near and distance, but the angle for near measures less, although it increases when either a) accommodative convergence or b) fusional convergence is reduced.
   a) The angle for near increases when a +3.00 lens is placed in front of each eye (simulated distance exotropia with high AC/A ratio)
   b) The angle for near increases when one eye is occluded (simulated distance exotropia with normal AC/A ratio).

Each of these manoeuvres should be performed to identify whether the exotropia is true or simulated, as true and simulated distance exotropia require different surgical approaches (Figure 6.1).

DIFFERENTIAL DIAGNOSIS

- Decompensated exophoria

MANAGEMENT

Non-surgical treatment

- Correct any refractive error
- Orthoptic exercises to improve convergence or reduce suppression may be useful

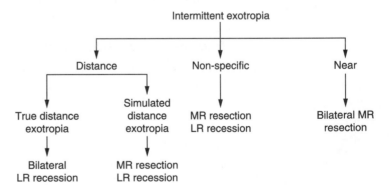

In those with lateral incomitance–reduce the LR recession by 1 mm

Figure 6.1 Surgical management of intermittent exotropia

- Careful monitoring of the strabismus for any signs of deterioration (see below) is essential

Surgical treatment Not all distance exo-deviations require surgical intervention and remain stable. Deciding on the optimum time for surgery can be difficult, but is usually when there is evidence of deterioration such as:

- Poor control of the deviation (manifest for >50% of the time, poor recovery on cover test or reduced BVA)
- Deteriorating stereoacuity
- Increase in the size of the deviation.

Surgical procedures: (Table 6.1 and Figure 6.1)

1. True divergence excess – symmetrical bilateral lateral rectus recessions
2. Simulated divergence excess (either normal or high AC/A ratio) – unilateral lateral rectus recession and medial rectus resection

In cases with lateral incomitance the amount of surgery to the lateral rectus should be reduced by 1 mm, and, if this is insufficient to correct the angle of deviation, then the surgery should be spread over three muscles – doing a smaller amount to each.

The aim is to slightly overcorrect the deviation in the immediate post-operative period (by 10–15 dioptres). This may lead to diplopia which can be very symptomatic for the patient in the short term, but there is usually gradual improvement. In patients with persistent symptoms or those who progress to develop amblyopia, treatment with occlusion, bifocal spectacles or prisms may be required. In some instances which persist, treatment with botulinum toxin or surgery is required (see Chapter 5 – consecutive esotropia).

Table 6.1 Exotropia – a guide to surgical treatment

Angle of squint	Bilateral LR recessions	or	LR recession/MR resection	
20D	5 mm		5 mm	4 mm
30D	6.5 mm		6.5 mm	5 mm
40D	8 mm		8 mm	5 mm
50D	9.5 mm		9 mm	5.5 mm

a) These measurements are only for concomitant deviations, with no underlying muscle or neurological pathology or previous surgery
b) The measurements for recessions are taken from the insertion of the muscle
c) The measurements should be altered based on the surgeon's personal results
d) If the horizontal angle is greater for near than distance relatively more should be done to the medial rectus than the lateral rectus, and vice versa
e) For angles >50 dioptres perform surgery to more than 2 horizontal recti
f) Exotropias with lateral incomitance require 1mm less recession to the lateral rectus
g) Aim to overcorrect consecutive and secondary exotropias

Intermittent exotropia (near)

There is an intermittent exotropia that occurs for near. This may be due to a low AC/A ratio or may be associated with poor fusional convergence.

CLINICAL FEATURES

- Intermittent exotropia for near, often with diplopia, exophoria for distance (near angle measures at least 10 dioptres more than the distance angle).
- Onset usually in late teens or early adult life.
- Headaches and vague asthenopic symptoms stimulated by close work.
- Equal visual acuities.
- Limited binocular function, with poor convergence.
- Concomitant, but may demonstrate lateral incomitance.
- May deteriorate with time to become constantly manifest.

DIFFERENTIAL DIAGNOSIS

- Convergence insufficiency

MANAGEMENT

Non-surgical management
- Correct any myopia
- Convergence exercises
- Base in prisms

Surgical management (Table 6.1 and Figure 6.1)   Indications for surgical intervention are the presence of a large angle or lack of response to conservative treatment.

- For small angles (<15 dioptres) a unilateral medial rectus resection is advisable
- For angles >15 dioptres, bilateral, symmetrical medial rectus resections
- Use adjustable sutures if possible, but note that these patients may be difficult to adjust as they tend to overconverge at the time of the adjustment and this may ultimately lead to an undercorrection. In all cases there is a risk of overcorrection for distance – but this usually settles with time

The aim of surgery is a functional result, with binocular vision for near and distance.

Intermittent exotropia (non-specific)

This is very similar to a distance exotropia (see above).

CLINICAL FEATURES

- Intermittently manifest exotropia for near and distance (angle equal for near and distance).
- Onset in early life (6–18 months).
- Tendency to close one eye in bright light.
- Good stereoacuity, but reduced motor fusion.
- Dense suppression when manifest, but amblyopia rare.
- Concomitant, but may demonstrate lateral incomitance (angle of deviation decreases on lateral gaze).
- Refractive error rare.
- May deteriorate with time to become constantly manifest.

MANAGEMENT

Non-surgical management
- Correct any refractive error
- Orthoptic exercises to improve convergence or reduce suppression may be useful
- Many remain stable, but careful monitoring of the strabismus for any signs of deterioration is essential (as for distance exotropias – see above)

Surgical treatment (Table 6.1 and Figure 6.1)
- Recession of the lateral rectus and resection of the medial rectus in the eye that most commonly deviates (see Chapter 12)
- In cases with lateral incomitance the amount of surgery to the lateral rectus should be reduced by 1mm and if this is insufficient to correct the angle of deviation then spread the surgery over three muscles.

The aim of surgery is to restore some degree of binocular vision for near and distance.

Exophoria (decompensating)

Exophoria is a latent divergent squint. Binocular single vision is achieved by adequate positive fusional vergence (the motor ability to converge). Exophoria is asymptomatic in the majority of people, but may decompensate and become symptomatic. Decompensation usually occurs spontaneously, but may be precipitated by a change in refractive

Table 6.2 Differentiating features between an intermittent exotropia and a decompensating exophoria

	Intermittent exotropia	*Decompensating exophoria*
Age at presentation	Usually early life	Any age – rarely the very young
Symptomatic	No	Yes
Suppression	Yes – dense	No
Binocular function	Motor and sensory defects	Motor defect, sensory function normal
Motor fusion range	Variable – often not reproducible	Reduced positive motor fusion range
Response to treatment	Limited	Good

status or spectacle correction, by excessive visual demands or by ill health. Exophoria becomes commoner with increasing age and may become symptomatic with the correction of presbyopia.

CLINICAL FEATURES

- Gradual, vague onset of symptoms (unless onset due to a sudden precipitant, e.g. change of glasses, head injury).
- Age of onset anytime – children or adults, but commoner in adults.
- Symptoms variable, e.g. eye strain, headache, blurring of vision, intermittent diplopia, closure of one eye for visually demanding activities.
- Equal vision.
- Cover test reveals reduced rate of recovery of exophoria (recovery absent in fully decompensated cases).
- BVA reduced.
- Reduced or absent positive motor fusion range (the ability to overcome base out prisms).
- Evidence of sensory fusion, with no suppression.
- Angle of deviation usually larger for near or for distance:
  - larger for near (near exophoria, with symptoms for close work)
  - larger for distance (distance exophoria, with symptoms for distance activities)
  - occasionally the angle may be equal for near and distance (non-specific exophoria), but this is unusual.
- Symptoms tend to occur with increased visual demand for the distance of maximal deviation.

DIFFERENTIAL DIAGNOSIS (TABLE 6.2)

- Primary intermittent exotropia

MANAGEMENT

Non-surgical treatment Treatment is offered if the decompensating/decompensated exophoria produces symptoms (see Chapter 12).

- Refraction – ensure that the most appropriate prescription is prescribed
- Orthoptic treatment – exercises to improve the positive fusional amplitude and convergence excercises
- Base in prisms – not recommended as a long-term solution as the requirement for prisms tends to increase gradually with the passage of time, but can be useful in elderly or unwell patients. Always use the smallest size of prism that relieves symptoms
- Botulinum toxin – injection of the lateral rectus muscle can be effective in reducing the angle of deviation and restoring binocular single vision; this, in turn, stimulates improvement in the motor fusion range and results in fewer symptoms and better control of the esophoria. This result is frequently long-standing, with beneficial effects long after the pharmacological effects of the toxin have worn off and may result in a cure of the condition (see Chapter 15).

Surgical treatment Surgery is recommended for patients who remain symptomatic despite appropriate conservative treatment. This is more likely to be required in those with large angled deviations and those that have responded badly to conservative measures.

Surgery should be carried out using adjustable sutures (Chapters 12 and 14) where possible and consists of:

- Bilateral medial rectus resections for near exophoria
- Bilateral lateral rectus recessions for distance exophoria
- Unilateral lateral rectus recession and medial rectus resection for non-specific exophoria.

The amount of surgery performed is based on the maximum angle of the deviation (see Table 6.1), bearing in mind that the aim of surgery is slightly to undercorrect the deviation.

Primary constant exotropia

This is the exotropic equivalent of early onset esotropia.

CLINICAL FEATURES
- Present from early life (<6 months).
- Usually alternating, but may be unilateral.
- Constant large angled exotropia present for near and distance.
- Binocular function usually absent.
- Refractive error rare.
- Associated with facial asymmetry and craniofacial abnormalities common.
- May develop DVD.

DIFFERENTIAL DIAGNOSIS
- Decompensated non-specific intermittent exotropia

MANAGEMENT
Non-surgical treatment Correct any refractive error, if present.

Surgical treatment (Table 6.1) Indications for surgery are on a cosmetic basis.

- Unilateral recession of lateral rectus and resection of medial rectus (see Chapter 12)
- Add in surgery to other eye if the angle >50 dioptres

The aim of surgery is slightly to overcorrect the angle to reduce the chance of re-divergence.

Secondary exotropia

CLINICAL FEATURES

- A divergent squint that develops because of loss of vision in the diverging eye.
- Poor visual acuity in the divergent eye.
- Concomitant.
- Commoner in adults (children tend to converge with reduced vision in one eye, although they tend to diverge as they grow older).

DIFFERENTIAL DIAGNOSIS

- Primary exotropia (see above)
- Consecutive exotropia (see below)

MANAGEMENT

Non-surgical management
- Investigate the cause of visual loss, if not known
- It may be possible to treat the cause of the loss of vision (e.g. remove a cataract, correct refractive error)
- The ipsilateral lateral rectus can then be treated with botulinum toxin, which will clarify the potential for binocular function
- In cases with binocular potential, toxin may restore binocular vision and no further treatment is required

Surgical management (see Table 6.1)   Surgical treatment is often needed on cosmetic grounds for those with poor vision that cannot be restored, or to restore binocular vision in those that are not responsive to conservative treatment.

- A lateral rectus recession and medial rectus resection should be performed on the poorly seeing eye (see Chapter 12)
- In adults, adjustable sutures should be used to get the best postoperative results (see Chapter 14)

The aim is slightly to overcorrect the deviation by up to 10 dioptres in cosmetic cases in order to provide long-term stability, or fully to correct the deviation in functional cases.

Consecutive exotropia

This is a divergent squint that occurs in a patient who previously had an esotropia. This may occur with or without surgical correction of the esotropia.

CLINICAL FEATURES

- Gradual onset exotropia (unless occurs in the immediate postoperative period – see complications, Chapter 16).
- Occurs at any age, but commonly early adult life.

- Weak or absent binocular function (motor and sensory fusion).
- Amblyopia common.
- Diplopia rare.
- History of previous esotropia (although some patients cannot remember their original deviation).
- If the patient has undergone surgical correction of the esotropia, scarring is usually visible over the insertions of the horizontal rectus muscles.
- Reduced adduction is common in the squinting eye, especially if surgery for the pre-existing esotropia has been carried out.
- An X or V pattern is common due to the eye swinging around a tight lateral rectus in such cases.

DIFFERENTIAL DIAGNOSIS

- Primary exotropia
- Secondary exotropia (the divergent eye may have reduced vision due to amblyopia)

MANAGEMENT

Non-surgical treatment

- Establish the likelihood of postoperative diplopia or BSV, using orthoptic tests
- If there is a risk of postoperative diplopia, botulinum toxin injection to the lateral rectus is used to straighten the squint temporarily and demonstrate whether the double vision is troublesome or ignorable

Surgical treatment (see Table 6.1) Surgery is usually performed for cosmetic reasons:

- Perform a lateral rectus recession and medial rectus advancement/ resection on the eye that is amblyopic or with the more restricted adduction (see Chapter 12)
- Use adjustable sutures where at all possible (see Chapter 14)
- Expose the medial and lateral rectus muscles before recessing or resecting, in order to determine the anatomy before performing the surgery
- In large angle deviations (>50 dioptres) surgery to the other eye may be indicated – patients should be informed about this as the decision may only be made after the start of surgery
- Sometimes there is a pseudo-tendon of scar tissue at the site of the old medial rectus insertion and care must be taken to ensure that the true medial rectus tendon has been found.

The aim is to overcorrect the angle of deviation (by up to 10 dioptres, depending on cosmetic appearances) to reduce future re-divergence. It is also useful to induce some degree of abduction weakness for the same reason.

Further reading

Bietti RB, Bagolini B. Problems related to surgical overcorrection in strabismus surgery. *J Pediatr Ophthalmol* 1965; **2**: 11–14

Bradbury JA, Doran RML. Secondary exotropia: a retrospective analysis of matched cases. *J Pediatr Ophthalmol Strabismus* 1993; **30**: 163–6

Jampolsky A. Differential diagnostic characteristics of intermittent exotropia and true exophoria. *Am Orthoptic J* 1954; **4**: 48–55

Lymburn EG, MacEwen CJ. Botulinum toxin in the management of heterophoria. *Br Orthoptic J* 1994; **51**: 38

Moore S. The prognostic value of lateral gaze measurements in intermittent exotropia. *Am Orthoptic J* 1969; **19**: 69–71

Pratt-Johnson JA, Barlow JM, Tilson G. Early surgery in intermittent exotropia. *Arch Ophthalmol* 1974; **84**: 689–94

Repka MX, Arnoldi KA. Lateral incomitance in exotropia: fact or artifact? *J Pediatr Ophthalmol Strabismus* 1991; **28**: 125

Scott WE, Keech RV, Marsh JA. The post-operative results and stability of exodeviations. *Arch Ophthalmol* 1978; **96**: 268–74

Wang FM, Chryssanthou G. Monocular eye closure in intermittent exotropia. *Arch Ophthalmol* 1988; **106**: 941

7

Vertical and pattern (A and V) deviations

This chapter examines:

Primary overaction of the superior and inferior oblique muscles

Dissociated vertical deviation (DVD)

Pattern deviations (A and V patterns)

Primary inferior oblique overaction

Primary overaction of the inferior oblique occurs when there is no evidence of weakness of the ipsilateral antagonist or the contralateral synergist.

CLINICAL FEATURES

- Elevation of the affected eye on adduction.
- No ipsilateral superior oblique or contralateral superior rectus weakness.
- Associated V pattern.
- Often bilateral but may be markedly asymmetrical.
- Negative Bielchowsky head tilt test.
- Commonly associated with early onset esotropia, although it may develop months to years after presentation.

Differential diagnosis

- DVD (see below)
- IV nerve palsy (ipsilateral)
- Superior rectus palsy (contralateral)

MANAGEMENT

Non-surgical treatment
- The inferior oblique overaction tends to become less obvious as children grow up and can be left untreated if it is purely a cosmetic problem

Surgical treatment Surgical intervention is indicated if the associated V pattern or vertical deviation is a) interfering with the development of binocular vision or b) causing a cosmetic problem.

- Weaken the inferior oblique muscle (recess or disinsert) – see Chapter 13
- If bilateral inferior oblique overaction is present, both inferior obliques should be weakened even if the condition is highly asymmetrical (unilateral surgery may be sufficient if surgery is carried out to non-fixing eye)
- If combined with surgery to correct esotropia, this should not influence the amount of horizontal rectus muscle surgery to be carried out

Dissociated vertical deviation (DVD)

This is a variable up-drift of the non-fixing eye, occurring when the patient is not concentrating fully. The patient is usually unaware of the movement, but it may be obvious to observers. There is a strong association with early onset esotropia. This is probably a supranuclear disorder, possibly a mechanism to suppress latent nystagmus.

CLINICAL FEATURES

- Slow up-drift and excyclotorsion of the non-fixing eye, which is densely suppressed.
- Slow recovery movement, in which the eye returns to the primary position by dipping slightly below the midline and intorting.
- Usually bilateral but often asymmetrical.
- The other eye does not deviate during the process.
- Asymptomatic (dense suppression during the movement).
- Age of onset in childhood, in association with a horizontal squint.
- Provoked by cover of the deviating eye.
- A head tilt may be present.

DIFFERENTIAL DIAGNOSIS

- Inferior oblique overaction (primary or secondary to IV nerve palsy): this may coexist and the two can be difficult to distinguish from one another

Helpful methods of differentiation between DVD and inferior oblique overaction are (NB they commonly co-exist):

- *Position of gaze:* **increased elevation in adduction which becomes less marked on abduction suggests inferior oblique overaction rather than DVD, which has no preference for the position of horizontal gaze**

- *A or V pattern:* **presence of a V pattern suggests inferior oblique overaction, an A pattern is more common in DVD**
- *Torsion:* **obvious excyclotorsion on elevation suggests DVD**
- *Hypotropia of other eye:* **by making the elevating eye fix in adduction. In inferior oblique overaction the other eye should depress under cover, in DVD (which is almost always bilateral to some extent) the other eye should elevate under cover**
- *Nystagmus:* **presence of latent nystagmus suggests DVD**

MANAGEMENT

Non-surgical treatment
- Treatment is for cosmetic purposes, therefore a non-surgical approach is preferable for those with small, cosmetically acceptable deviations. In some patients, the DVD becomes less obvious with time, although adults can present *de novo* when the unsightly appearance begins to bother them
- In very asymmetric cases it may be possible to promote fixation with the eye with more deviation by fogging the other eye by increasing or reducing the spectacle prescription

Surgical treatment Surgery is indicated for cosmetic purposes. Even with surgery, the deviation often returns in the long term although not as markedly.

Surgery should always be bilateral, even in very asymmetrical cases. Surgery is directed towards disabling upgaze:

- Superior rectus recessions of between 8 and 12 mm on hang back sutures to avoid placing sutures near the superior oblique tendon (see Chapter 12)
- Anteriorization of the inferior obliques (see Chapter 13). The latter is especially useful when DVD and inferior oblique overaction coexist, but is now the procedure of choice in DVD alone as this produces a better result with long-term stability.

Primary superior oblique overaction

Superior oblique overaction is usually a primary event as inferior oblique weakness is not common, although it may occur secondary to bilateral recessions of the inferior recti. It may be due to an abnormally sagittal insertion of the superior oblique tendon and is common in craniofacial dysostoses in which there is probably excyclorotation of the whole orbit.

CLINICAL FEATURES
- Depression of the affected eye in adduction.
- There may be a vertical deviation in the primary position, although this is unusual.

- No evidence of ipsilateral inferior oblique weakness or contralateral inferior rectus weakness.
- Coexistent A pattern, which may result in a compensatory head posture.
- Usually bilateral.
- It may be associated with a horizontal deviation.

MANAGEMENT

Non-surgical treatment   Many patients with superior oblique overaction have minimal symptoms and treatment is not considered.

In craniofacial dysostoses surgery is not likely to be profitable due to the abnormal muscle anatomy.

Surgical treatment   Intervention is indicated if the overaction:

- becomes symptomatic due to the development of an abnormal head posture
- threatens binocular vision.

Surgery consists of posterior tenotomy of the superior oblique, usually bilaterally (see Chapter 13).

A pattern

This is a pattern of squint in which the horizontal deviation becomes more esotropic on upgaze and more exotropic on downgaze (so that the pattern of the squint resembles the letter **A**). The underlying cause may be:

- Oblique muscle dysfunction – superior oblique overaction/inferior oblique weakness
- Vertical rectus dysfunction – inferior rectus weakness (palsy or secondary to surgery)
- Horizontal muscle dysfunction – abnormal insertion or action of the medial/lateral recti (secondary to surgery or spontaneously).

CLINICAL FEATURES

- The squint in the primary position may be an esotropia or an exotropia. The difference in deviation is considered significant if the horizontal angle varies by more than 10 dioptres between upgaze and downgaze.
  - A esotropia: a convergent squint which increases in angle on upgaze and decreases on downgaze
  - A exotropia: a divergent squint which increases in angle on downgaze and decreases on upgaze

- The patient may adopt a compensatory head posture (usually chin up with A esotropia and chin down with A exotropia) to reduce size of the horizontal deviation.

MANAGEMENT

Non-surgical treatment Small deviations which are non-symptom producing do not require any treatment.

Surgical treatment If the A pattern is symptom producing, either by inducing an abnormal head posture to maintain binocular vision, or by interfering with maintenance of binocular function – surgery is the treatment of choice.

Surgical procedure depends on underlying cause (Figure 7.1):

1. Oblique muscle dysfunction – superior oblique overaction/inferior oblique weakness
   - posterior tenotomy of the superior oblique (if there is no oblique dysfunction do *not* weaken superior oblique) (see Chapter 13)

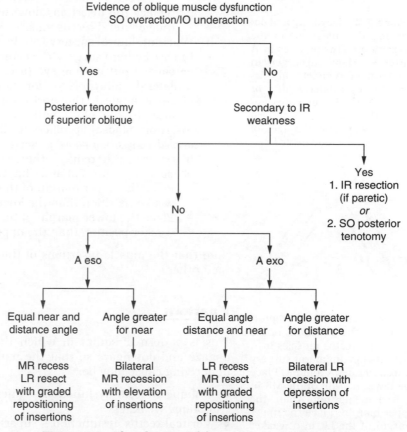

Figure 7.1 Flow diagram of the management of A patterns

2. No oblique dysfunction present and inferior rectus function reduced
   - Consider strengthening the inferior rectus if this will not induce a deviation in the primary position or in downgaze (e.g. in inferior rectus palsy)
   - Superior oblique posterior tenotomy is the treatment of choice *only* when this is not possible (e.g. in thyroid cases where the IR is surgically weakened and there is no vertical deviation in the primary position – this situation can be prevented by moving the inferior rectus medially during recession) (see Chapter 12)
3. No oblique dysfunction present and inferior rectus function normal: surgery should be carried out to the horizontal rectus muscles and this may be combined with recession +/- resection of these muscles to treat any associated eso- or exotropia in the primary position:
   a) When surgery to both eyes is to be performed:
   - Elevate or depress the positions of medial or lateral rectus insertions (see Figure 7.2 and Chapter 12)
     - An A eso pattern – recess both medial recti and move the insertions upwards towards the superior rectus (the medial rectus is always moved towards the apex of a pattern)
     - An A exo pattern – recess both lateral rectus muscles and replace the insertions downwards towards the inferior rectus (move lateral rectus muscles away from the apex of a pattern)
   b) When unilateral surgery is to be performed:
   - In cases where surgery to correct the horizontal strabismus is to be carried out on one eye (a recess/resect procedure because of unilateral amblyopia or for squints that have equal near and distance angles), the horizontal rectus muscles should be re-sutured to the globe with the upper and lower parts of the insertion placed at different distances from the limbus. This *graded re-positioning* is preferred to elevating or depressing the insertions as it reduces the risk of inducing unwanted torsion effects (see Figure 7.3 and Chapter 12)
     - Place the upper margin of the medial rectus in a preferentially weaker position than the lower margin
     - Place the lower margin of the lateral rectus in a preferentially weaker position than the upper margin.

Note that the muscle insertions of the same eye are always parallel to each other.

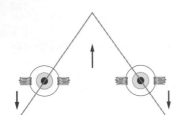

Figure 7.2 Elevating and depressing the insertions of the horizontal rectus muscles in A patterns for bilateral surgery in the form of symmetrical surgery to contralateral MRs or LRs. Move MRs upwards towards the apex of the pattern or LRs away from the apex of the pattern (i.e. downwards)

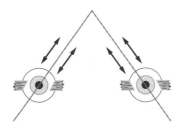

Figure 7.3 Graded repositioning of the insertions of the horizontal rectus muscles in A patterns for unilateral surgery to ipsilateral MR and LR. Place the lower margin of the MR in a weaker position than the upper margin. Place the upper margin of the LR in a weaker position than the lower

V pattern

This is pattern of squint in which the horizontal deviation alters on upgaze and downgaze so that the pattern resembles the letter V. The underlying cause may be:

- Oblique muscle dysfunction – inferior oblique overaction/superior oblique weakness
- Vertical rectus dysfunction – superior rectus weakness/tight inferior rectus (often associated with thyroid eye disease)

- Horizontal muscle dysfunction – abnormal insertion or action of the medial/lateral recti (secondary to surgery or spontaneously).

CLINICAL FEATURES

A V pattern is considered significant if the difference in the horizontal deviation is 15 dioptres or more in upgaze compared with downgaze.

- V esotropia is a horizontal convergent strabismus in which the angle of squint increases on downgaze and decreases on upgaze.
- V exotropia is a divergent squint in which the angle of squint reduces on downgaze and increases on upgaze.
- The patient may adopt a compensatory head posture (usually chin up with V exotropia or chin down with V esotropia).

MANAGEMENT

Non-surgical treatment   Commonly V patterns do not require any treatment, unless they become symptom producing or cosmetically unacceptable. They may become less obvious with the passage of time.

Surgical treatment   The surgical procedure carried out depends on the underlying cause:

1. Oblique muscle dysfunction – inferior oblique overaction/superior oblique weakness
   - Weaken the inferior oblique (disinsert or recess) (see Chapter 13)
2. No oblique dysfunction present and a tight inferior rectus present:
   - recess the inferior rectus on adjustable sutures (if this is possible without inducing a deviation in the primary position or in downgaze) (see Chapter 12)
   - laterally transpose the inferior rectus half to one muscle width
3. No oblique or vertical rectus dysfunction present:
   Surgery should be carried out to the horizontal rectus muscles and this may be combined with recession +/− resection of these muscles to treat any eso- or exotropia in the primary position:
   a) When surgery to both eyes is to be performed:
   - Elevate or depress the positions of medial and lateral rectus insertions (see Figure 7.4 and Chapter 12)
     - V eso pattern – recess both medial rectus muscles by the appropriate amount for the horizontal deviation and move the insertions downwards towards the inferior rectus (the medial rectus is always moved towards the apex of the pattern)
     - V exo pattern – recess both lateral recti by the appropriate amount from the horizontal deviation and move the lateral rectus muscles upwards (the lateral recti move away from the apex of the pattern)
   b) When unilateral surgery is to be performed:
   - In cases where surgery to correct the horizontal strabismus is to be carried out on one eye (a recess/resect procedure because of unilateral amblyopia or for squints that have equal near and

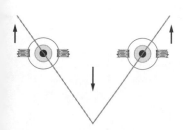

Figure 7.4   Elevating and depressing the insertions of the horizontal rectus muscles in V patterns for bilateral surgery in the form of symmetrical surgery to contralateral MRs or LRs. Move MRs downwards towards the apex of the pattern or LRs away from the apex of the pattern (i.e. downwards)

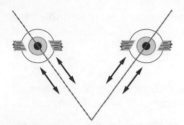

Figure 7.5 Graded repositioning of the insertions of the horizontal rectus muscles in V patterns for unilateral surgery to ipsilateral MR and LR. Place the lower margin of the MR in a weaker position than the upper margin. Place the upper margin of the LR in a weaker position than the lower

distance angles), the horizontal rectus muscles should be resutured to the globe with the upper and lower parts of the insertion placed at different distances from the limbus. This *graded re-positioning* is preferred to elevating or depressing the insertions as it reduces the risk of inducing unwanted torsion effects (see Figure 7.5 and Chapter 12)

– Place the lower margin of the medial rectus in a preferentially weaker position then upper margin
– Place the upper margin of the lateral rectus in a preferentially weaker position than the lower margin

Further reading

Burke JP, Scott WE, Kutschke PJ. Anterior transposition of the inferior oblique muscle for dissociated vertical deviation. *Ophthalmology* 1993; **100**: 245–50

Fink WH. The A & V syndrome. *Am Orthop J* 1959; **9**: 105

Guyton DL, Weingarten PE. Sensory torsion as the cause of primary oblique muscle overaction/underaction and A- and V-pattern strabismus. *Binoc Vision Eye Muscle Surg Q* 1994; **9** (Suppl.): 209–36

Jampolsky A. Oblique muscle surgery of the A and V pattern. *J Pediatr Ophthalmol* 1965; **2**: 31

Matthews TD, Patel BCK, Lee JP, Fells P. Disinsertion and recession of the inferior oblique muscle. *Proceedings of the 6th Meeting of the International Strabismological Association*, Brussels, 1992

Mein J, Johnson F. Dissociated vertical divergence and its association with nystagmus. In: Mein J, Moore S. (eds). *Orthoptics, research & practice*, Kimpton, London. 1981; 14–16

Scott WE, Drummond GT, Keech RV. Vertical offsets of horizontal recti muscles in the management of A and V pattern strabismus. *Aust NZJ Ophthalmol* 1989; **17**: 281

Scott WE, Sutton VJ, Thalacker J. Superior rectus recessions for dissociated vertical deviation. *Ophthalmology* 1982; **89**: 317–322

Urist MJ. The etiology of the so-called A and V syndromes. *Am J Opthalmol* 1958; **46**: 835–44

8

Palsies of the ocular motor nerves

This chapter examines:

III nerve palsy

IV nerve palsy

VI nerve palsy

These may occur individually or in combination. Each is discussed individually.

III nerve palsy

The superior division of the III nerve supplies the superior rectus and the levator palpabrae superioris muscle; the inferior division supplies the medial rectus, the inferior rectus, the inferior oblique muscle and the pupil. The nucleus of the III nerve is complex as it supplies so many muscles. The superior rectus is supplied by the contralateral nucleus, the levator is supplied bilaterally by a common nucleus and the other muscles are supplied by the ipsilateral nucleus.

CLINICAL FEATURES

a) Total palsy
  - a large exotropia with a small hypotropia, intorsion
  - reduced adduction, elevation and depression of the affected eye
  - ptosis
  - fixed and dilated pupil
  - face turn to opposite side (if no ptosis)
  - overaction of contralateral synergists
b) Partial palsy may affect one or any combination of the extraocular muscles and the lid and the pupil may or may not be involved
  - the superior or inferior divisions may be affected independently
    - *superior division* – superior rectus and levator palpabrae
    - *inferior division* – inferior rectus, inferior oblique, medial rectus and pupil

- each individual muscle may be involved (all are fairly rare)
  - *Medial rectus* – weakness of adduction. Differentiate from an internuclear ophthalmoplegia (abducting nystagmus may be present in both conditions, but convergence is usually preserved in an internuclear ophthalmoplegia)
  - *Inferior rectus* – weakness of depression, especially in abduction
  - *Inferior oblique* – weakness of elevation in adduction. Differentiate from Brown's syndrome by the forced duction test
  - *Superior rectus* – weakness of elevation. Often asymptomatic. Needs to be differentiated from a contralateral IV nerve palsy as with spread of concomitance the two conditions may appear similar. Helpful methods of differentiation include:

Table 8.1 Differentiating features between superior rectus and contra-lateral superior oblique weakness

	Superior rectus weakness	*Superior oblique weakness*
Eye movements	Reduced elevation in abduction	Reduced depression in adduction
Pattern	V pattern	A pattern
Near/distance	Vertical angle > for distance	Vertical angle > for near
AHP	Chin up	Chin down
Bielchowsky test	Negative	Positive

AETIOLOGY

- Congenital – rare
- Microvascular disease (associated with diabetes, hypertension or atherosclerosis)
- Aneurysm of the posterior communicating artery (usually painful)
- Demyelination
- Trauma (including neurosurgical trauma)
- Intracranial infection or inflammation
- Neoplasia – primary or secondary

DIFFERENTIAL DIAGNOSIS

The diagnosis is usually straightforward, but:

- Myasthenia gravis may mimic a III nerve palsy, especially if a ptosis is present
- Blow out fracture may mimic the vertical movements, limit the medial rectus and cause a traumatic mydriasis

MANAGEMENT

Non-surgical treatment
1. Initial management
   - Full neurological examination – examine all the cranial nerves with particular emphasis on the adjacent IV and VI nerves
     - IV nerve – ask the patient to abduct the eye and look down. Observe for any incyclotorsion

- VI nerve – ask the patient to abduct the eye
  (it is difficult to examine for the IV nerve if the VI is also damaged, but it is usually possible to identify some torsion, by observing movement of the conjunctival blood vessels, if the IV is intact)
- Investigate – primary presentations of non-traumatic III nerve palsy should be investigated in all patients
  - Microvascular screen
  - Neuroimaging
  - *A painful palsy involving the pupil suggests a posterior communicating artery aneurysm and requires* emergency *neurosurgical referral*
- Alleviate diplopia (if the ptosis does not cover the pupil). Occlusion is usually necessary due to the incomitance and size of the deviation, although temporary prisms or botulinum toxin may be useful in partial palsies
- Await spontaneous recovery; those due to microvascular disease usually recover, but other causes are less likely to do so. (Recovery from a III nerve palsy may produce aberrant regeneration, especially after trauma or aneurysm surgery. It does not occur in microvascular lesions. This commonly affects the upper lid with elevation of the ptosis on depression or adduction, or the pupil with pupillary constriction associated with adduction. This may produce a confusing clinical picture.)

2. Long-term management
   - A non-surgical approach is an option because of the complexity of the eye movement disorder and the limited expected outcome. Possible management includes:
     - No treatment (ptosis prevents diplopia)
     - Occlusive spectacle lens, contact lens or intraocular lens may be considered in those in whom the ptosis has lifted, but the extraocular muscle imbalance persists
     - In some of those with partial recovery a prism may be usefully incorporated into the glasses

Surgical treatment
- As surgical treatment may be complex with a limited outcome it must not be undertaken lightly. Surgery should not be considered until there has been a stable period of at least 4–6 months
- In those who wish surgery the eye movements should be repaired prior to lid surgery to elevate the ptosis

1. Total, unrecovered III nerve palsy: this is difficult to treat successfully, as so many muscles are not functioning. The aims, limitations and possible outcomes of surgery must be fully explained as the optimum result is likely to be a compromise as the surgeon can do no more than improve the cosmesis in the primary position, but the movements of the eye will be very poor. There will probably be no useful binocular function as lack of eye movements in the affected eye ensure a very limited motor fusion range. An occlusive contact lens or intraocular lens may be required, even once the eye has been placed in the optimum position.

Table 8.2 Isolated muscle involvement in III nerve palsy (other muscles unaffected)

	Partial involvement or recovery	*Complete unrecovered*
MR	Recess ipsilateral LR Resect ipsilateral MR (adjustable sutures)	Medial transposition of IR and SR (resect each by 5 mm)
IR	Recess ipsilateral SR	1. Inferior transposition of LR and MR 2. Recess ipsilateral SR, as a 2nd stage (if 1 not enough) 3. Recess/Faden contralateral IR to increase field of BSV
SR	1. Recess ipsilateral IR Resect ipsilateral SR (adjustable sutures) 2. Weaken contralateral IO	Leave alone, unless hypotropia in primary position – if present: 1. Recess ipsilateral IR (adj.) 2. Transpose MR and LR upwards
IO (rare)	Rarely requires treatment	1. Post-tenotomy of ipsilateral SO 2. Recess contralateral SR (adjustable sutures)

Surgical correction of a total, unrecovered III should consist of surgery to the affected eye:

- a massive lateral rectus recession on a hang back suture (as far as it will go – usually 12–15 mm) and a huge medial rectus resection (as much as is possible – usually up to 10 mm) (see Chapter 12)
- the insertions of each horizontal rectus muscle should be supra-placed when sutured to the globe
- stay sutures are placed through the insertions of the superior and inferior rectus muscles and passed through the upper lid at the medial canthus to hold the eye in adduction and elevation for up to 6 weeks (see Chapter 12)

2. Partial palsy (or partial recovery) (Table 8.2)
- There is a better chance of regaining some useful, although often limited, binocular function in partial cases
- Surgery depends on the pattern of paresis
- Assess binocular potential as some patients lose the ability to fuse
- The surgical approach depends on the pattern of motility disturbance, however the following principles apply:
  - Recess the overacting ipsilateral antagonists to optimize the movements of the affected eye, this may be supplemented by a resection of the partially recovered muscle, which may help to balance the ocular position, although this depends upon the degree of muscle function
  - Where there is no recovery of muscle function, transposition surgery is recommended (see Chapter 12)
  - Recess the contralateral synergists, as this may improve the synchronicity of movement of the two eyes and improve the field of BSV

– Surgery should always be carried out using adjustable sutures as the results are unpredictable (see Chapter 14)

Treatment for different types of partial third nerve palsy:

- *Superior division* – surgical approach is the same as superior rectus (see Table 8.2)
- *Inferior division* – surgical approach is similar to total III nerve palsy (see above)
- *Individual muscle involvement* – (see Table 8.2). Weakness of the inferior rectus requires treatment to reduce diplopia in downgaze, even if there is no deviation in the primary position. Superior rectus weakness only requires treatment if there is a manifest deviation in the primary position.

IV nerve palsy

The IV nerve supplies the superior oblique muscle. Superior oblique palsy is relatively common.

CLINICAL FEATURES

- History of vertical diplopia with or without tilting (or torsion) of the images
- Compensatory head posture
  - a head tilt toward the opposite shoulder, face turn towards the unaffected eye, with slight chin depression (unilateral cases)
  - chin down (bilateral cases)
- A vertical deviation in the primary position that increases when the eyes move away from the hypertropic (affected) side
- A positive three step test with Bielchowsky positive (see Chapter 1)
- Patients with a congenital IV nerve palsy may have a head tilt present in old photographs and it is worth asking the patient to bring some in if this is suspected
- The pattern of eye movement abnormality varies as IV nerve palsy has a number of different clinical patterns:
  - Predominately inferior oblique overaction is the commonest presentation, i.e. elevation of the affected eye on adduction with minimal superior oblique weakness
  - Predominately superior oblique weakness, i.e. poor depression of the affected eye on adduction with only minimal inferior oblique overaction (rarer presentation)
  - Poor depression of the affected eye which has the appearance of a 'double depressor palsy'
  - Torsion: this is most commonly a problem with bilateral cases – there may be little to see on eye movements but torsion measurements are significant, especially on downgaze

It is important to recognize these patterns as in each case the management is different (Figure 8.1).

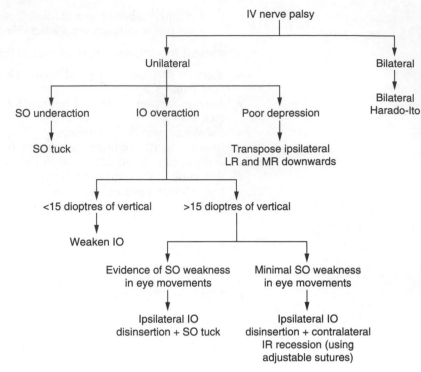

Figure 8.1 IV nerve palsy

Always suspect IV nerve palsies to be bilateral, as they may be very asymmetrical, and the less obvious side easily overlooked. Be especially suspicious in the following circumstances:

- **Aetiology – closed head injury**
- **Patient complains of torsion as a major feature**
- **Torsion measures >12 degrees (in primary position, increasing on depression)**
- **V eso pattern to the eye movements**
- **Chin down head posture**
- **Left over right deviation on dextro-version which reverses to a right over left on laevo-version**
- **Alternating hypertropia on Bielchowsky head tilt test, i.e. positive to both sides**

AETIOLOGY

Congenital
- The majority of IV nerve 'palsies' are congenital in origin although they may only present in adulthood when they 'decompensate'. These may be due to an abnormality of the muscle tendon rather than a defect of the nerve supply

Acquired
- Severe closed head injury damages the IV nerve as it exits from the mid-brain (almost always bilateral)
- Microvascular disease in association with atherosclerosis, diabetes or hypertension
- Mid-brain disease, rarely (which usually has associated brain-stem clinical findings)

Differentiation between the congenital and acquired IV nerve palsies
- **Onset – usually vague for congenital cases**
- **Symptoms – usually lack of symptoms for congenital cases, despite large vertical deviation**
- **Torsion is usually not a feature of congenital cases**
- **Vertical fusion range – usually large in congenital cases**
- **Congenital cases often have intermittent suppression**
- **Congenital cases often have a degree of facial asymmetry**
- **Childhood photos often show an abnormal head tilt – prior to symptoms being evident**

DIFFERENTIAL DIAGNOSIS

- Primary inferior oblique overaction associated with childhood esotropia
- DVD
- Contralateral superior rectus weakness (see above under III nerve palsy)

MANAGEMENT

Non-surgical treatment   Initial management
- Full history and neurological examination – this should differentiate the congenital cases from the acquired
- Investigate if the aetiology is considered to be acquired
  - Microvascular screen
  - Neurological imaging in those with other neurological symptoms or signs, or those <40 years
- Alleviate diplopia if present (patching is often required because of the torsion)
- Await recovery if the aetiology is acquired

Surgical treatment   Most patients with symptoms from IV nerve palsies require surgical treatment.
   The surgical treatment depends on:

- the pattern of extraocular imbalance
- the vertical fusion range: (it is always better to leave the vertical deviation undercorrected and surgery should be tailored to correct the amount of the deviation that requires to be corrected rather than the size of the deviation).

Surgical options consist of (Figure 8.1):

1. Predominately inferior oblique overaction:
   - Disinsert the inferior oblique (Chapter 13). This will correct between 12 and 15 dioptres of height in the primary position as well as reducing the elevation in adduction
     - if >15 dioptres of height needing correction in primary position, with minimal or no weakness of the superior oblique on testing eye movements, perform a contralateral inferior rectus recession using adjustable sutures in addition (see Chapter 14) (remember the deviation may measure more than 15 dioptres, but it is the amount of this that needs to be corrected that is important - beware of overcorrection)
     - if >15 dioptres of height needing correction in primary position and there is evidence of superior oblique weakness on testing eye movements, perform an ipsilateral superior oblique tuck in addition (see Chapter 13)
2. Predominately superior oblique weakness:
   - Carry out a superior oblique tuck (Chapter 13)

   The aim is to provide depression in adduction, without inducing a Brown's syndrome.
3. Poor depression of the affected eye:
   - Transfer the medial and lateral recti downwards (inverse Knapp procedure – Chapter 12)

   The aim is to provide a better downward movement.
4. Torsion:
   - Perform a Harado-Ito procedure (Chapter 13) – usually bilateral

   The patient may take a few days to adjust to the new position of the eyes after this procedure.

VI nerve palsy

VI nerve palsy affecting the function of the lateral rectus muscle is the commonest acquired palsy affecting an ocular motor nerve.

CLINICAL FEATURES

- Esotropia which increases on looking towards the affected side
- Reduction of abduction of the affected eye
- Deviation greater for distance than for near
- A head turn may develop towards the affected side
- If the palsy is mild, the diagnosis may only be made by turning the patient's face away from the affected side and getting them to fixate a distant target, as this increases the esodeviation.

AETIOLOGY

Children
- Congenital
- Benign viral illness

- Trauma
- Hydrocephalus
- Brain-stem pathology

Adults
- Microvascular disease (hypertension, diabetes, atherosclerosis)
- Closed head trauma
- Intracranial or nasopharyngeal tumours
- Demyelination

DIFFERENTIAL DIAGNOSIS

- Habitual lateral rectus weakness in long-standing esotropia
- Duane's syndrome
- Mobius syndrome
- Thyroid eye disease with tight medial recti
- Myasthenia gravis

MANAGEMENT

Non-surgical treatment   Initial management
- Clinical examination and investigations: establish the underlying diagnosis by taking a history and performing a thorough neuro-examination, examining the long tracts and other cranial nerves carefully, especially looking for papilloedema. All children should have neuroimaging, even though benign VI nerve palsy is the commonest cause in childhood. In adults who have no other signs or symptoms, do a microvascular screen, but no other imaging is required unless other features develop
- Alleviate diplopia/face turn, while awaiting spontaneous recovery which will take place in over 80% of cases
  - using prisms, patching or by injecting botulinum toxin into the ipsilateral medial rectus. (Toxin should only be used in the early phase if the diagnosis is absolutely clear)
  - in children, amblyopia should be prevented by alternating occlusion or by injecting botulinum toxin into the ipsilateral medial rectus under ketamine anaesthesia to promote binocular vision until recovery takes place

Later treatment

- In those who do not wish or are not suitable for surgical intervention, treat with occlusion, prism or toxin

Surgical treatment   In cases where there is not a full recovery of eye movements, surgical correction should be considered after a stable period lasting 4–6 months.

The first step is an injection of botulinum toxin into the ipsilateral medial rectus, as this will determine the degree of recovery of the lateral rectus and therefore what surgical procedure is required (Figure 8.2).

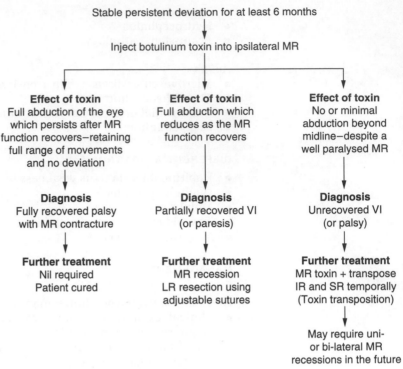

Stable persistent deviation for at least 6 months

Inject botulinum toxin into ipsilateral MR

Effect of toxin	**Effect of toxin**	**Effect of toxin**
Full abduction of the eye which persists after MR function recovers–retaining full range of movements and no deviation	Full abduction which reduces as the MR function recovers	No or minimal abduction beyond midline–despite a well paralysed MR
Diagnosis	**Diagnosis**	**Diagnosis**
Fully recovered palsy with MR contracture	Partially recovered VI (or paresis)	Unrecovered VI (or palsy)
Further treatment	**Further treatment**	**Further treatment**
Nil required Patient cured	MR recession LR resection using adjustable sutures	MR toxin + transpose IR and SR temporally (Toxin transposition)

May require uni-
or bi-lateral MR
recessions in the future

Figure 8.2   VI nerve palsy

- If there is full abduction while the medial rectus is weak, due to the action of the botulinum toxin, and this is maintained after the toxin has worn off and the medial rectus function recovers, this indicates a *fully recovered palsy with medial rectus contracture*
  - The injection of botulinum toxin can result in a permanent cure and no further treatment may be required An ipsilateral medial rectus recession should be performed, on adjustable sutures, if there is any residual angle
- If full, or almost full, abduction occurs while the medial rectus is weak, but the deviation returns as the medial rectus recovers, then this indicates a *partial recovery of the lateral rectus*
  - Surgical treatment involves a large ipsilateral medial rectus recession combined with a lateral rectus resection using adjustable sutures

  The aim of surgery is to centralize the field of binocular vision and to regain a good range of extraocular movements
- If there is no (or minimal) abduction beyond the midline when the medial rectus is weak, then a total, or *unrecovered palsy* is diagnosed
  - Transposition of the superior and inferior rectus muscles laterally should be performed while the medial rectus remains paralysed (see Chapter 12) (or repeat the injection at a future date 1–2 weeks before scheduled surgery)

  The aim of surgery is an immediate overcorrection, with the patient being slightly divergent. As the toxin wears off this divergence should become less. It is possible that one or both medial recti may require to be weakened at a later date when the toxin has worn off and the anterior segment circulation has recovered.

Further reading

Ellis FD, Helveston EM. Superior oblique palsy: diagnosis and classification. *Int Ophthalmol Clin* 1976; **16**: 127–35

Fitzsimmons R, Lee JP, Elston J. Treatment of sixth nerve palsy in adults with combined botulinum toxin chemodenervation and surgery. *Ophthalmology* 1998; **95**: 1535–42

Hermann JS. Masked bilateral superior oblique paresis. *J Pediatr Ophthalmol Strabismus* 1981; **18**: 43–8

Knapp P. Classification and treatment of superior oblique palsy. *Am Orthop J* 1974; **24**: 185–90

Knapp P, Moore S. Diagnosis and surgical options in superior oblique surgery. *Int Ophthalmol Clin* 1976; **16**: 137–49

Kraft SP, Scott WE. Masked bilateral superior oblique palsy. *J Pediatr Ophthal Strabismus* 1986; **23**: 264–72

Lee JP. Modern management of sixth nerve palsy. *Aust NZ J Ophthalmol* 1992; **20**: 41–6

Lee JP, Gregson RMC. Traction sutures in the management of fixed divergent strabismus. In: Kaufmann H (ed.) *Transactions of the 21st ESA Meeting, Salzburg* 1993; 397–9

Lee JP, Harris S, Cohen J, Cooper K, MacEwen CJ, Jones S. Results of a prospective randomised trial of botulinum toxin therapy in acute unilateral sixth nerve palsy. *J Pediatr Ophthalmol Strabismus* 1994; **31**: 283–6

Mitchell PR, Parks MM. Surgery for bilateral superior oblique palsy. *Ophthalmology* 1982; **89**: 484–8

Morris RJ, Scott WE, Keech RV. Superior oblique tuck surgery in the management of superior oblique palsies. *J Pediatr Ophthalmol Strabismus* 1992; **29**: 337–46

Moster ML, Savino PJ, Sergott RC, Bosley RM, Schatz NJ. Isolated sixth nerve palsies in younger adults. *Arch Ophthalmol* 1984; **102**: 1328–30

Murgatroyd H, Fleming I, MacEwen CJ. Reduced adduction following lateral transposition of the vertical rectus muscles for sixth nerve palsy. *Br Orthoptic J* 2002; **59**: 30–2.

Noonan CP, O'Connor M. Surgical management of sixth nerve palsy. *Br J Ophthalmol* 1995; **79**: 431–4

Price NC, Vickers S, Lee JP, Fells P. The diagnosis and surgical management of acquired bilateral superior oblique palsy. *Eye* 1987; **1**: 78–85

Riordan-Eva P, Lee JP. Management of VIth nerve palsy – avoiding unnecessary surgery. *Eye* 1992; **6**: 386–90

Schumacher-Reero LA. Yoo KW. Solari FM. Biglan AW. Third cranial nerve palsy in children. *Am J Ophthalmol* 1999; **128**: 216–21

Simons BD. Surgical management of ocular motor cranial nerve palsies. *Sem Ophthalmol* 1999; **14**: 81–94

Tiffin PAC, MacEwen CJ, Craig EA, Clayton G. Acquired palsy of the oculomotor, trochlear and abducens nerves. *Eye* 1996; **10**: 377–84

Restrictive disorders

> The following conditions will be covered in this chapter:
>
> **Thyroid eye disease**
>
> **Blow out fractures**
>
> **Strabismus following retinal detachment surgery**
>
> **Myopic restrictive strabismus**

Restrictive disorders often demonstrate unique features for each patient, although certain commoner patterns of abnormality occur. Complex management strategies are beyond the scope of this text, but broad principles of treatment are given (Table 9.1), with some commonly recognized patterns of extraocular motility imbalance being highlighted.

Thyroid eye disease

This is an autoimmune orbitopathy which is associated with autoimmune thyroid disease. Fifty percent of patients with autoimmune thyroid disease will develop evidence of thyroid eye disease. In the vast

Table 9.1 Principles of surgical management in restrictive strabismus

- Identify which muscles are weak and which are restricted (forced duction test/ raised intraocular pressure)
- Always recess restricted muscles – resection may cause further reduction in movement
- Always use adjustable sutures – the results are highly unpredictable
- Improve movements in ipsilateral eye first by recessing overacting ipsilateral antagonists
- Balance the eyes by recessing contralateral synergists
- Problems on downgaze need careful evaluation and treatment
- Horizontal deviations require recession of the medial rectus (esotropia) or the lateral rectus (exotropia)
- Problems on upgaze can usually be left untreated (if no vertical deviation in the primary position)

majority this is a minor condition and only a small group develop significant problems which threaten vision or cause symptoms of extraocular muscle disturbance. It may produce a restrictive type of ocular motility disturbance.

Thyroid eye disease consists of two phases. The extraocular muscles become infiltrated with inflammatory cells causing swelling and stiffness of the muscles in the first, inflammatory phase. In the second, cicatricial stage the muscles become fibrotic, scarred and tight. The disease can affect any of the extraocular muscles, but tends to affect the inferior rectus most commonly followed by the medial rectus, the superior rectus and lastly the lateral rectus. Involvement of the oblique muscles does not give rise to clinical signs.

CLINICAL FEATURES

In both phases there are similar clinical findings, which vary in severity from very mild to severe.

- Commonly bilateral condition, but may be very asymmetrical
- Red, irritable eyes
- Upper lid retraction
- Lid lag
- Proptosis
- Restriction of eye movements

Phase 1 (inflammatory phase)   The features above are accompanied by evidence of inflammation and changing signs.

- Swelling – lid swelling, chemosis, caruncle swelling, proptosis (which may be progressive)
- Redness – conjunctival injection, lid redness
- Pain – on eye movements, generalized pain behind the eyes
- Reduced function – restriction in eye movements which may be progressive, optic nerve dysfunction due to compression by the enlarging muscles

Phase 2 (cicatricial phase)

- Features of inflammation reduce (i.e. less swelling, redness, discomfort)
- Condition becomes more stable
- Any restriction of eye movements stabilizes

Some patients present in Phase 2 (commonly young women with thyroid eye disease) and do not appear to have had clinical evidence of an active Phase 1.

Extraocular muscle imbalance   Any eye movement disorder can occur in thyroid eye disease as any muscle can be involved. There is, however, a common pattern of muscle involvement which causes restriction in movement when the eye is *moved away* from the involved muscles. The following are the most recognized patterns of muscle involvement:

- *Restriction of upgaze* – due to a tight inferior rectus is the commonest motility disorder observed. This may present as a unilateral hypotropia, due to unilateral or markedly asymmetrical inferior rectus involvement. Alternatively, in cases with bilateral, symmetrical involvement, this presents as a chin up compensatory head posture. Patients with tight inferior recti have a V pattern with an exotropia on elevation
- *Restriction of abduction* – due to medial rectus involvement, is the next most common. This presents as an esotropia, with reduced abduction (it may simulate a VI nerve palsy)
- *Combination of vertical and horizontal restriction* – due to inferior rectus and medial rectus contracture (which may be unilateral or bilateral). This presents as a combination of the defects in restriction of upgaze and restriction of abduction
- *Restriction of depression* – due to involvement of the superior rectus, causing a hypertropia with limitation in depression. Superior rectus involvement may occur with inferior rectus muscle involvement and it is essential to examine a full range of movements, particularly upgaze and downgaze

Sensory changes

- Patients commonly develop an enlarged vertical fusion range, due to the slow development of the deviation
- Patients commonly develop an abnormal head posture to maintain single vision

MANAGEMENT

Initial management

- Clinical examination – the diagnosis can often be made on clinical grounds alone on the basis of typical signs
- Investigation – evidence of thyroid dysfunction (thyroid function tests, thyroid antibodies) is common (either past or present), but not universal
- MRI scanning of the orbit demonstrates enlarged muscles and is helpful in differentiating between the inflammatory and cicatricial phases using the STIR sequence – in the former there is oedema of the rectus muscles which appear bright white in colour

Non-surgical treatment

- Stabilize thyroid functions if patient presents with abnormal thyroid functions
- Alleviate diplopia– patching, prisms or promotion of an abnormal head posture
- In the inflammatory phase
    - Monitor optic nerve function
        - Fields of vision
        - Colour vision (Ishihara plates)

- Monitor eye movements (including uniocular fields of fixation (UFOFs), Hess charts and fields of BSV)
- Monitor clinical activity of the disease (Mourits score or other)
- Botulinum toxin may be useful in reversing the deviation in this phase
- Systemic immunosuppression (steroids or other agents) or local immunosuppression (orbital radiotherapy) may be helpful in progressive cases. It is likely, but not proven, that aggressive immunosuppression during the active, inflammatory phase of the disease reduces the need for corrective strabismus surgery later

- In the cicatricial phase immunosuppression is contraindicated and the management is with prisms if the deviation is small, or with surgery if the deviation is large. Botulinum toxin has no role in this phase

Surgical treatment

- Surgery should only be considered when the condition has moved into the cicatricial stage and is stable
- If orbital decompression is being considered, this should be carried out prior to extraocular muscle surgery
- Lid surgery should take place following strabismus surgery
- Always recess muscles – do not resect (see Table 9.1)
- Use adjustable sutures (see Table 9.1)

1. Restriction of upgaze – due to inferior rectus involvement
   Surgical management:
   - Inferior rectus recession using adjustable sutures (one or both eyes)
     - Replace the recessed inferior rectus muscle medially to reduce the likelihood of the development of a postoperative A pattern (see Chapter 12)
     - Leave the vertical deviation undercorrected
     - Recessions of more than 3 mm will result in retraction of the lower lid
2. Restriction of abduction – (one or both eyes)
   Surgical management:
   - Medial rectus recession using adjustable sutures (see Chapter 14)
   - Both medial recti should be recessed if there is any evidence of bilateral involvement, even in those with small angles of deviation
3. Combined horizontal and vertical deviations – abduction and elevation deficit, with horizontal and vertical deviations
   - Surgical management – medial and inferior rectus recessions using adjustable sutures (see Chapter 14)
4. Restriction of depression
   - Surgical management – superior rectus recession using adjustable sutures (see Chapter 14)

Aims of surgery The disease process may lead to significant restriction of movement and therefore it is possible that the patient will not regain a full field of binocular single vision. The aim is to maximize the field of

BSV in the primary position, to each side and in downgaze. Upgaze should be sacrificed if it is not possible to retain a full field of BSV. Always leave vertical deviations undercorrected or there will be a reversal of the deviation in the medium to long term.

Blow out fracture

CLINICAL FEATURES

- There is a history of blunt trauma to the affected eye, or face in the region of the orbital rim
- Diplopia is usually apparent immediately after this incident (although this may be delayed by closure of the eyelids due to swelling)
- There are a number of patterns of ocular motility defects which are recognized after a blow out fracture, although any vertical or horizontal deviation is possible depending on the pattern of injury:
  - Limitation of downgaze
  - Limitation of upgaze
  - Limitation of upgaze and downgaze, causing a reversal of the vertical deviation from upgaze to downgaze
  - The eye may be hypotropic, hypertropic or straight in the primary position
- Eye movements show a 'restrictive' limitation of the eye, as indicated by no, or minimal, overaction of the ipsilateral antagonist muscles
- Other features include:
  - enophthalmos of the affected eye
  - loss of sensation affecting the infraorbital area.

AETIOLOGY

- Incarceration of orbital fibrous septae in the orbital floor fracture site
- Incarceration of the inferior rectus muscle in an orbital floor fracture site
- Haemorrhage or oedema of the inferior rectus
- Muscle ischaemia – causing weakness of the inferior rectus
- Nerve palsy – due to damage to the nerve supply of the inferior rectus

(To differentiate between weakness and restriction – see Chapter 1.)

MANAGEMENT

Initial management

- Examine the patient's ocular motility defect as soon as possible after the injury has taken place, ensuring to document:
  - The size of the deviation
  - Hess chart
  - Field of BSV

Review 5–7 days later to identify any change in the condition

- Examine eye to ensure that no significant ocular damage has taken place
- CT scanning of the orbits should be performed if surgery is being considered

Non-surgical treatment

- Observation – the majority of ocular motility disturbances associated with blow out fractures resolve spontaneously with time
- Prisms are rarely useful due to the incomitant nature of the strabismus

Surgical treatment   Surgery to the orbital floor is considered if there is:

- Diplopia in the primary position or in downgaze which persists beyond one week to 10 days after the injury
- Evidence of entrapment (positive forced duction test, increase of intraocular pressure on upgaze of >5 mm and/or radiological evidence of entrapment)
- A large fracture on radiological examination
- Persistent significant enophthalmos at 10–14 days after injury.

Surgery to the orbital floor is commonly undertaken in cooperation with ENT or maxillofacial surgeons. If indicated this should take place 10–14 days after the injury, a period that gives time for spontaneous improvement to take place, but is not long enough for significant scar tissue to develop.

The surgical approach to the extraocular muscles depends on the pattern of motility disorder (Figure 9.1).

- This depends on the position of the eyes in the primary position and on the pattern of ocular limitations.
- Leave at least 6 months, often longer (there may be no change at all for several months) and ensure that the deviation is stable.
- A forced duction test must be performed in all cases to identify the pattern of passive restriction.

Surgical options consist of (Figure 9.1):

1. *Deviation in the primary position*   Due to a restricted inferior rectus – causing a hypotropia with limited elevation.

- Recession of the inferior rectus (adjustable sutures) (see Chapters 12 and 14).

The aim is to improve the ocular position in the primary position, but not to induce a hypertropia in downgaze. This requires careful adjustment.

2. *Limitation of downgaze*   Due to inferior rectus palsy. The surgical treatment depends on the deviation in the primary position and on the degree of depression deficit:

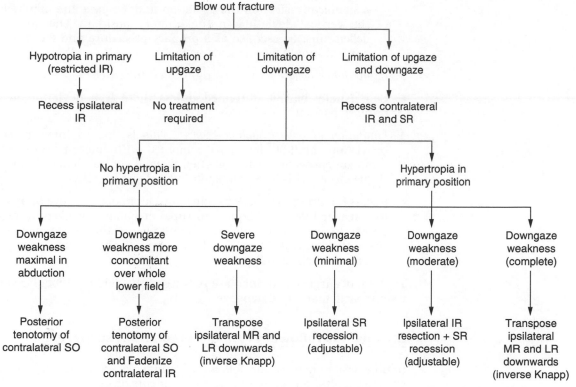

Figure 9.1 Blow out fracture – management of ocular motility imbalance

- Minimal or no vertical deviation in the primary position (aim to improve downgaze without inducing a vertical deviation)
  - If the downgaze deficit is incomitant, being maximal in downgaze on abduction – carry out a posterior tenotomy of the contralateral superior oblique muscle (see Chapter 13)
  - If the downgaze deficit is more concomitant over the whole lower field – Fadenize the contralateral inferior rectus in addition to the superior oblique posterior tenotomy to balance the lower field (see Chapter 12)
  - If the downgaze deficit is severe – transpose the lateral and medial recti inferiorly (see Chapter 12). This commonly does not induce a vertical deviation, but if it does this can be corrected later.
- Hypertropia in the primary position:
  - With a minimal downgaze deficit – carry out an ipsilateral superior rectus recession using adjustable sutures (see Chapters 12 and 14)
  - With a moderate downgaze deficit – resect the ipsilateral inferior rectus in addition to the ipsilateral superior rectus recession using adjustable sutures (see Chapters 12 and 14)
  - With a complete downgaze deficit – transpose the lateral and medial rectus muscles inferiorly (see Chapter 12) – this will have

a significant effect on the deviation in downgaze and may reduce the vertical deviation in the primary position. The downgaze deficit must be rectified as a primary procedure and any residual vertical should be corrected later.

3. *Limitation of upgaze* Due to a tight inferior rectus.

● Can usually be left untreated unless there is a deviation in the primary position.

4. *Limitation of upgaze and downgaze* This is due to inferior rectus restriction (limited elevation) combined with inferior rectus palsy (limited depression). There is often a small central field of binocular single vision. This is very difficult to treat successfully.

● Recess inferior and superior rectus muscles in opposite eye (may need to consider inferior oblique and superior oblique weakening procedures also, depending on the incomitance of the deviation and on the pattern of restriction). Such patients are often not keen to have surgery to their 'good' eye.

The aim of surgery is to increase the size of the field of binocular single vision, particularly in downgaze.

Strabismus following retinal detachment surgery

Double vision may occur following retinal detachment surgery, due either to limitations of extraocular movements or sensory changes. This may, or may not, be troublesome and frequently settles given time.

CLINICAL FEATURES
● The patient complains of diplopia shortly after retinal detachment surgery
● The eye movements may demonstrate reduced ductions in one or more directions depending on the underlying problem
● Any deviation may be horizontal, vertical or torsional

AETIOLOGY
Diplopia after retinal detachment surgery may occur because of alterations in the rotations of the globe or because of sensory changes. These factors must be carefully considered and their relative effects assessed before any surgical procedure is contemplated.

The underlying cause must be identified, as surgical treatment is not always recommended. Causes include:

● Restrictions of one or more movements due to trauma to the Tenon's capsule or to one or more of the extraocular muscles at the time of surgery
● The pressure of an explant on one or more of the extraocular muscles
● The breakdown of a pre-existing phoria, following a period of reduced vision in one eye

- The inability to fuse images caused by alteration in the macular architecture (pucker, scarring) creating barriers for fusion
- Central loss of fusion
- Anisometropia, due to surgically induced refractive errors.

MANAGEMENT

Non-surgical treatment

- Observation – commonly spontaneously improves or patients develop suppression
- Careful refraction – with prescription of glasses or contact lenses
- Botulinum toxin may be used to try to realign the eyes temporarily and to diagnose whether fusion is possible by reducing the size of the squint. This may result in a permanent realignment if fusion is strong enough and the restrictions to movement only minimal
- Prisms are useful in those with small deviations
- If straight in the primary position the best option may be to leave alone

Surgical treatment

- A forced duction test must be performed to identify the pattern of passive restriction
    - Adhesions should be divided and a recession of the affected muscle performed (using adjustable suture) (see Chapter 14)
- Reduce the overaction of the contralateral agonist. (Patients are often reluctant to undergo surgery on their fellow eye)
    - This may be done in the short term using botulinum toxin injection
    - In the long term by recession (adjustable) or Faden of the overacting contralateral synergist
- Removal of external plombage should only be performed with the consent of the retinal surgeon. Improvements in the ocular rotations are not usually found following plomb removal

The aim of surgery is to regain single vision in the primary position and to maximize the field of binocular single vision.

Myopic restrictive strabismus

In large, highly myopic eyes, the lateral rectus can flip, usually downwards, over the enlarged globe, reducing the function of the lateral rectus and causing the eye to rotate upwards or downwards.

CLINICAL FEATURES
- High myopia
- Large angled convergent strabismus
- Reduced abduction (active and passive restriction)
- Variable vertical deviation, often with upshoots and downshoots

- Potential for binocular vision
- Develops in adult life

DIFFERENTIAL DIAGNOSIS

- Thyroid eye disease
- VI nerve palsy

MANAGEMENT

Surgical treatment (Table 9.1)   Treatment is surgical.

- A medial rectus recession should be performed using adjustable sutures (see Chapter 14)
- Resection of the lateral rectus is *contraindicated*, as this would compound the situation

Further reading

Ballantyne L, MacEwen CJ. Blow out fractures; What happens to ocular motility after repair of the fracture? *Br Orthoptic J* 1999; **56**: 58–60

Bagshaw J. Heavy eye phenomenon. *Br J Ophthamol* 1996; **23**: 73

Bahn RS, Heufelder AE. Pathogenesis of Graves' ophthalmopathy. *N Engl J Med* 1993; **329**: 1468–75

Demer JL, von Noorden GK. High myopia as an unusual cause of restrictive motility disturbance. *Surv Ophthalmol* 1989; **33**: 281

Dulley B, Fells P. Long-term follow up of orbital blow-out fractures with an without surgery. *Mod Probl Ophthalmol* 1975; **14**: 467–70

Fells P, McCarry B. Diplopia in dysthyroid eye disease. *Trans Ophthalmol Soc UK* 1986; **105**: 413

Fells P, Kousoulides L, Pappa A, Munro P, Lawson J. Extraocular muscle problems in thyroid eye disease. *Eye* 1994; **8**(5): 497–505

Fison PN, Chignell AH. Diplopia after retinal detachment surgery. *Br J Ophthalmol* 1987; **71**: 521–5

Goel R, Crewdson J, Chignell AH. Astigmatism following retinal detachment surgery. *Br J Ophthalmol* 1983; **67**: 327–9

Lee JP, Page B, Lipton J. Treatment of strabismus after retinal detachment surgery with botulinum neurotoxin A. *Eye* 1991; **5**: 451–5

Lipton JR, Page AB, Lee JP. Management of diplopia on downgaze following orbital trauma. *Eye* 1990; **4**: 535–7

Lyons CJ, Vickers S, Lee JP. Botulinum toxin in dysthyroid strabismus. *Eye* 1990; **4**: 538–42

McCarry B, Fells P, Waddell E. Difficulties in the management of orbital blow-out fractures in patients under 20 years old. In: Revault AP, Lenk M (eds). *Transactions of the Fifth International Orthoptic Congress*. LIPS, Lyon. 1984; 283

Howarth F, Dewar JA, MacEwen CJ. Radiotherapy in thyroid eye disease: possible beneficial effect on the orthoptic status of patients. *Br Orthoptic J* 2000; **57**: 59–64

Maurino V, Kwan ASL, Lee JP. Review of the inverse Knapp procedure: indications, effectiveness and results. *Eye* 2001; **15**: 7–11

Mourits MP, Van Kempen-Harteveld ML, Garcia MBG, Koppeschaar HPF, Tick L, Terwee CB. Radiotherapy for Graves' orbitopathy: randomised placebo-controlled study. *Lancet* 2000; **355**: 1505–9

Mourits RW, Prummel MF, Wiersinge WM, Koorneef L. Measuring eye movements in Grave's ophthalmopathy. *Ophthalmology* 1994; **101**: 1341

Munox M, Rosenbaum AL. Long-term strabismus complications following retinal detachment surgery. *J Pediatr Ophthalmol Strabismus* 1987; **24**: 309

Prummel MF, Mourits MP, Blank L et al. Randomized double-blind trial of prednisone versus radiotherapy in Graves' ophthalmology. *Lancet* 1993; **342**: 949–54

Putterman AM, Stevens T, Urist MJ. Non-surgical management of blow-out fractures of the orbital floor. *Am J Ophthalmol* 1974; **77**: 232–9

Rubin ML. The induction of refractive errors by retinal detachment surgery. *Trans Am Ophthalmol Soc* 1975; **73**: 452–90

Sewell JJ, Knobloch WH, Eifrig DE. Extraocular muscle imbalance after surgical treatment for retinal detachment. *Am J Ophthalmol* 1974; **78**: 321–3

Tallstedt L, Lundell G, Torring O et al. Occurrence of ophthalmopathy after treatment for Graves' hyperthyroidism. The Thyroid Study Group. *N Eng J Med* 1992; **326**: 1733–8

Waddell E, Fells P, Koorneef L. The natural and unnatural history of a blow-out fracture. *Br Orthoptic J* 1982; **39**: 29

10

Complex ocular
motility problems

> This chapter examines:
>
> **Brown's syndrome**
>
> **Duane's syndrome**
>
> **Mobius syndrome**
>
> **Double elevator palsy**
>
> **Congenital fibrosis of the extraocular muscles**
>
> These are complex, incomitant disorders of ocular motility due to congenital anomalies of the extraocular muscles, the nerve supply to the extraocular muscles, or of the orbital anatomy.

Brown's syndrome (or superior oblique tendon sheath syndrome, SOTSS)

This is a congenital or, rarely, acquired abnormality which limits movement of the superior oblique tendon through the trochlea.

CLINICAL FEATURES

- Inability to elevate the affected eye in adduction, either actively or passively (may have difficulty elevating the eye in direct elevation and even in abduction in marked cases)
- Usually unilateral
- Usually no deviation in the primary position (either horizontal or vertical)
- Minimal muscle sequelae (overaction of the contralateral superior rectus may be present)
- A 'click' may be present on palpation of the trochlear region when the patient is asked to move the eye upwards and downwards in adduction
- Abnormal head posture – chin up with face turn away from the affected eye

DIFFERENTIAL DIAGNOSIS

- Inferior oblique palsy
- Double elevator palsy
- Congenital fibrosis of the extraocular muscles
- Motility defect secondary to orbital trauma

MANAGEMENT

Non-surgical treatment

- Most cases will spontaneously resolve and should be observed. The presence of the 'click' (which is palpated over the area of the trochlea as the eye moves from upgaze to downgaze) is a good prognostic sign for spontaneous resolution.
- In acquired inflammatory cases (e.g. in association with rheumatoid arthritis) steroid injection into the region of the trochlea is said to be helpful and surgery is not indicated

Surgical treatment Surgery should only be carried out if the Brown's syndrome is causing a hypotropia in the primary position, there is evidence that binocular vision in the primary position is being compromised or it is inducing the adoption of a significant head posture.

- Superior oblique tenotomy nasal to the superior rectus muscle (see Chapter 15). At surgery passive elevation of the eye in adduction should be attempted and repeated after the superior oblique tenotomy to confirm that elevation in adduction is much freer. Despite this the Brown's pattern will persist after the surgery but should gradually disappear in the majority of cases
- Superior oblique underaction commonly develops over the following months. This can be treated with an inferior oblique disinsertion if it becomes problematic

Duane's syndrome

Duane's retraction syndrome is a condition of varying severity in which there is anomalous innervation of the lateral rectus by the III cranial nerve, which contracts on adduction.

CLINICAL FEATURES

- Limitation of adduction, abduction or both
- Retraction of the globe on attempted adduction
- Narrowing of the palpebral fissure on attempted adduction and widening on attempted abduction
- Usually esotropic in the primary position (without AHP) but may be exo or straight
- Abnormal head posture – face turn in the direction of the most limited movement
- Upshoot or downshoot of the affected eye on adduction

- Diplopia rare, despite poor movements
- Reduced convergence
- Binocular single vision (BSV) in primary position with absence of diplopia on eye movements due to suppression on lateral gaze
- Limited muscle sequelae
- Bilateral or unilateral, but commonly asymmetric and considered 'unilateral'
- Various ocular and systemic abnormalities (all rare)

There are two classifications of the syndrome based on the pattern of horizontal movement abnormality and the deviation in the primary position. Patients may not be easily classified and the overall features of the syndrome need to be recognized (as above).

DIFFERENTIAL DIAGNOSIS

Diagnosis of the condition is usually straightforward.

- VI nerve palsy (should have a deviation in the primary position and no retraction)
- Scarred medial rectus from multiple previous operations
- Restrictive strabismus of high myopia
- Medial wall blow out fracture

MANAGEMENT

Non-surgical treatment   Most patients with Duane's syndrome require no treatment other than an explanation about the aetiology of the condition and the reassurance that surgery cannot produce normal movements in the affected eye. Children should be observed at regular intervals to ensure no loss of sensory fusion.

Surgical treatment   Surgery is rarely indicated, but it may be for:

1. a marked head posture
2. dealing with disfiguring up- and downshoots
3. severe retraction
4. loss of BSV in primary position

1. Abnormal or compensatory head posture   In *classical eso-Duane's* a head turn to the side of the affected eye is often adopted. This may be extreme and surgery indicated to relieve this. Surgical approach depends on the size of the deviation in the primary position and on the amount of reduction of abduction. The amount of surgery required is more than would be expected. Because of the poor adduction of the affected eye it is inadvisable to over recess the ipsilateral medial rectus, although it is possible to carry out a large recession to the contralateral medial rectus.

i)   When abduction is moderately reduced:
   - Recession of the ipsilateral medial rectus of 3 mm in deviations of up to 15 dioptres (see Chapter 12)

- Recession of ipsilateral medial rectus of 3 mm and contralateral medial rectus of 5 mm in deviations of 15–30 dioptres
- Recession of both medial rectus muscles – ipsilateral 5 mm and contralateral up to 10 mm in deviations of >30 dioptres
- *Resection of the lateral rectus should never be performed*

ii) When abduction is markedly reduced or absent:

- A transposition of the inferior and superior rectus muscles laterally to the insertion of the lateral rectus. This should be accompanied by an injection of botulinum toxin to the ipsilateral medial rectus
- If a medial rectus recession is subsequently required this should not exceed 3 mm, to prevent divergence

In *exo Duane's* adduction is reduced and there may be a face turn away from the affected eye. Surgery consists of an ipsilateral lateral rectus recession.

2. Upshoots and downshoots   These abnormal vertical movements occur due to the 'leash effect' of the lateral rectus as this tight muscle slides down or up over the equator of the globe. Surgery is aimed at preventing this from happening and can be done in a number of different ways:

- Recess the ipsilateral lateral rectus (see Chapter 12)
- A lateral rectus Faden (posterior fixation) suture of the ipsilateral lateral rectus (see Chapter 12).

The latter option is particularly useful if there is no horizontal squint in the primary position.

3. Globe retraction   Surgery for globe retraction alone is not usually indicated, but if the cosmetic problem is severe, this may be required.

- Recess the ipsilateral lateral rectus muscle at least 10 mm
- This may have to be combined with a recession of the medial rectus if there is an esotropia in the primary position (see Chapter 12).

4. Losing BSV in primary position   An increasing angle of squint which threatens binocular function is a similar problem to an increasing abnormal head posture, but has become manifest in a different manner. Treatment should follow the same lines (see head posture above).

Mobius syndrome

This is a congenital syndrome of bilateral VI, VII, IX and XII nerve palsies with associated systemic abnormalities.

CLINICAL FINDINGS

- Large angled esotropia, present since birth
- Bilateral abduction weakness
- Abnormal face turn, alternating to each side to take up fixation with either esotropic eye

- Amblyopia and significant refractive error uncommon
- Facial weakness on both sides of the face leading to:
  - a 'mask-like' face
  - poor eyelid closure (Bell's phenomenon intact)
  - swallowing and feeding difficulties
- Systemic abnormalities – a variety of such abnormalities have been recorded

DIFFERENTIAL DIAGNOSIS

- Congenital VI nerve palsy
- Early onset esotropia
- Duane's retraction syndrome

MANAGEMENT

Non-surgical management

- Ensure corneal protection
- Treat any refractive error and amblyopia

Surgical treatment Treat in the same way as an unrecovered VI nerve palsy by injecting the medial rectus with botulinum toxin and transposing the superior and inferior rectus muscles laterally (Chapters 8 and 12).

The aim of surgery is to improve the position of the eyes in primary position and to promote the development of binocular vision.

Double elevator palsy

This is an inability to look up with one eye probably caused by a congenital supranuclear abnormality of unknown aetiology. It may present as an acquired defect after mid-brain CVA.

CLINICAL FEATURES

- Inability to elevate one eye voluntarily, either in adduction, abduction or direct elevation
- Present since birth, but not always noticed until sitting up
- Usually uniocular
- May be associated with ptosis, or pseudo-ptosis
- Adoption of a chin up compensatory head posture to maintain binocular function
- Amblyopia may occur, depending on success of head posture
- Bell's phenomenon is usually intact
- Forced duction normal

DIFFERENTIAL DIAGNOSIS

The diagnosis is usually obvious, since Bell's phenomenon should be preserved.

- Brown's syndrome
- Tight inferior rectus
- Blow out fracture
- Superior division III nerve palsy

MANAGEMENT

Non-surgical treatment   Treat amblyopia, including prescription of refractive error, if any.

If the hypotropia is severe, surgery should be performed before amblyopia treatment is complete.

Surgical treatment

- Forced duction test to evaluate any tightness of the inferior rectus
- Vertical transposition of the horizontal recti upwards to the insertion of the superior rectus (Knapp procedure) (see Chapter 12)
- Inferior rectus recession, but only if there is contracture of that muscle felt on forced duction (see Chapter 12)
- Ptosis repair should be carried out later, if this is required

The aim of surgery is to improve the position of the eye in primary position, to relieve an abnormal head posture and to promote the development of binocular vision.

Congenital fibrosis of the extraocular muscles

This is a rare group of congenital diseases, in which there is progressive restriction of eye movements of unknown aetiology. There is fibrosis of the extraocular muscles with adhesions between the muscles, the conjunctiva and the eye.

CLINICAL FEATURES

- Usually bilateral, but may be very asymmetric
- Minimal movement of the affected eye(s)
- The affected eye is usually pulled into a position of downgaze and/or convergence and may be so severe that the cornea is not visible
- Chin up head posture
- Ptosis

DIFFERENTIAL DIAGNOSIS

- Congenital III nerve palsy
- Congenital myasthenia gravis
- Atypical Duane's syndrome
- Chronic progressive external ophthalmoplegia (CPEO)
- Double elevator palsy

MANAGEMENT

Non-surgical treatment Treat any refractive error and amblyopia (usually present in asymmetrical cases).

Surgical treatment Surgery is required in children with large head postures to improve the ocular deviation in primary position or for poor cosmesis. Any surgery for ptosis should take place after surgery to the extraocular muscles.

- Large recession of the affected muscles – usually the medial and inferior rectus – on long hang back sutures. Recess the conjunctiva to augment the result.

Aims of surgery: a full range of movements is not possible, but improvement in the primary position is possible and may reduce the head posture and improve cosmesis.

Further reading

Aylward GW, Lawson J, McCarry B, Lee JP, Fells P. The surgical treatment of traumatic Brown syndrome. *J Pediatr Ophthalmol Strabismus* 1992; **29**: 276–83

Cross HE, Pfaffenbach DD. Duane's retraction syndrome and associated congenital malformations. *Am J Ophthalmol* 1972; **73**: 442

Fells P, McCarry B. Surgical options in Duanes retraction syndrome. In: Lenk Schafer M, Calcutt C, Doyle M, (eds). *Orthoptic horizons. Transactions of the 6th International Orthoptics Congress.* 1987. British Orthoptic Society, London

Ficker LA, Collin JRO, Lee JP. Management of ipsilateral ptosis with hypotropia. *Br J Ophthlamol* 1986; **70**: 732–6

Gregerson E, Rindziunski E. Brown's syndrome – a longitudinal long-term study of spontaneous course. *Acta Ophthalmol* 1993; **71**: 371

Hansen E. Congenital general fibrosis of the extraocular muscles. *Acta Ophthalmol* 1968; **46**: 469

Leone CR, Leone RT. Spontaneous cure of congenital Brown's syndrome. *Am J Ophthalmol* 1986; **102**: 542

Parks MM, Brown M. Superior oblique tendon sheath syndrome of Brown. *Am J Ophthalmol* 1975; **79**: 82–6

Rogers GL, Bremer DL. Surgical treatment of the upshoot and downshoot in Duanes retraction syndrome. *Ophthalmology.* 1984; **92**: 1380–3

Rowe FJ, Wong ML, MacEwen CJ. Duane's retraction syndrome – bilateral until proven otherwise. *Br Orthoptic J* 1991; **48**: 36

von Noorden GK, Oliver P. Upshoot and downshoot in Duane's syndrome. *J Pediatr Ophthalmol Strabismus* 1986; **23**: 212

von Noorden GK, Murray E. Superior oblique tenectomy in Brown's syndrome. *Ophthalmology* 1982; **89**: 303

11

Nystagmus

This chapter examines how surgery or botulinum toxin to the extra-ocular muscles may help to reduce symptoms in some forms of nystagmus.

Nystagmus is a condition that rarely benefits from surgical treatment to the extraocular muscles. However, under certain circumstances extra-ocular muscle surgery may help a few patients with some forms of nystagmus. Congenital nystagmus is most likely to benefit from surgical intervention.

Congenital nystagmus

This is an abnormal movement of the eyes that usually begins within the first 6 months of life.

CLINICAL FEATURES
- Bilateral involuntary oscillatory movements of the eyes
- Usually horizontal movements
- Always uniplanar
- Waveform may be complex to maximize foveation
- Null zone, which may lead to the adoption of a compensatory head posture
- Dampens on convergence
- Reduced visual acuity (variable)
- No oscillopsia

DIFFERENTIAL DIAGNOSIS
Other forms of acquired nystagmus.

MANAGEMENT
Non-surgical treatment

- Refraction, commonly associated refractive error

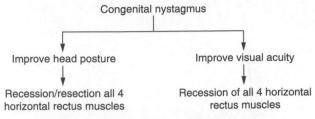

Figure 11.1 Aims of surgery for nystagmus

- Observation is the usual line of treatment, as the patients are frequently asymptomatic and the condition tends to improve with time
- Contact lens wear can help to dampen the nystagmus and hence improve the visual acuity

Surgical treatment Aims of surgery for nystagmus (Figure 11.1):

1. To reduce a compensatory head posture where this is unacceptable
2. To improve visual acuity, by reducing oscillopsia.

1. Head posture
Compensatory head postures occur in nystagmus because of the existence of a 'null-point', which is the position of gaze in which the nystagmus is most dampened. The null-point is the position of gaze in which visual acuity is best (Figure 11.2a–c).

PROCEDURES

Face turn right/left Surgery involves recessions and resections of the rectus muscles of both eyes, in order to realign the eyes within the orbits, without inducing a deviation (Figure 11.2d) (Kestenbaum or the so-called 5,6,7,8 procedure Table 11.1). This procedure produces a deviation of the eyes in the direction of the head turn, and therefore helps to straighten the head (Figure 11.2a–f).

For those with large head postures, the amount of surgery can be increased to up to 40% more than suggested above, but it is important to increase the amount to each muscle by the same percentage.

In those with super-added strabismus, the amount of surgery to be carried out to correct the squint should simply be added to the amount required for correction of the head posture.

Chin-up/down Vertical head postures are trickier to improve surgically but essentially a recession–resection procedure of the vertical recti is required on both sides. Again, the eyes are moved in the direction of the head posture: each eye undergoes symmetrical and equal surgery (Table 11.2).

The patient must be warned about the possible effects of lower lid retraction or elevation by the inferior rectus surgery.

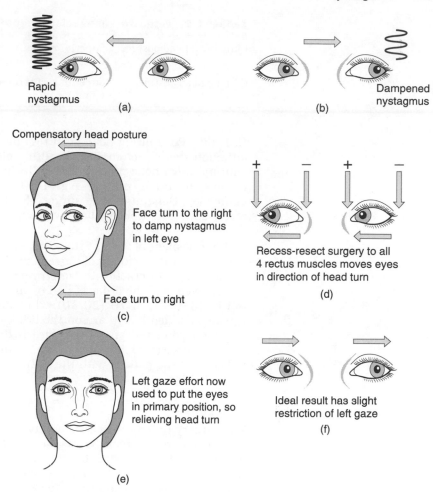

Figure 11.2 Nystagmus. (a) When eyes look to the right the nystagmus increases; (b) The nystagmus dampens on left gaze; (c) Face turn to the right to damp nystagmus in left gaze; (d) recess–resect surgery to all four muscles moves eyes in direction of head turn; (e) left gaze effort now used to put eyes in primary position, so relieving head turn; (f) ideal result has slight restriction of left gaze

Table 11.1 Horizontal rectus muscle surgery to correct head posture

Head turn right	Right medial rectus recession 6 mm	Right lateral rectus resection 7 mm	Left medial rectus resection 5 mm	Left lateral rectus recession 8 mm
Head turn left	Right medial rectus resection 5 mm	Right lateral rectus recession 8 mm	Left medial rectus recession 6 mm	Left lateral rectus resection 8 mm

Table 11.2 Vertical rectus muscle surgery to correct head posture

| Chin down head posture | Superior rectus recessions 8 mm | Inferior rectus resections 4 mm |
| Chin up head posture | Superior rectus resections 6 mm | Inferior rectus recessions 6 mm |

Head tilt   Pure tilting head postures due to nystagmus are uncommon, although there is often a small tilting element to a head turn or to a chin-up/down head posture. Head tilts in patients with nystagmus may be due to other causes, e.g. DVD or congenital oblique muscle anomalies. Oblique muscle surgery for head tilts due to nystagmus is rarely done and probably best avoided.

2. Improvement of visual acuity

Reduction of the velocity of movement is associated with an increase in visual acuity. In practice the improvement of the visual acuity that can be achieved is of the order of half of one standard Snellen line, i.e. from 6/12 (20/40) to 6/10 (20/30). This modest improvement may be of benefit to patients who are on the brink of the driving standard. In the UK the driving test visual standard is the equivalent of 6/10 (20/30) and so surgery to improve visual acuity to permit driving is only indicated if the patient with the nystagmus is *already* very close to this level of vision.

PROCEDURES

The surgery to improve visual acuity consists of very large recessions of all four horizontal recti by 10 mm. Little restriction of eye movement appears to be produced by this procedure, but the change in the nystagmus is immediate and a cosmetic bonus if the improvement in acuity is less than the patient expects.

Nystagmus blockage esotropia

This is an early onset esotropia due to active convergence being used to dampen congenital nystagmus. The esotropia develops in patients with congenital nystagmus in order to enhance monocular acuity by damping the nystagmus using convergence (see Chapter 5).

Acquired nystagmus

There are a variety of different types of acquired forms of nystagmus commonly secondary to neurological disease. Affected patients are usually very symptomatic due to oscillopsia and reduced visual acuity. There are specific and non-specific forms, each with different clinical features, the description of which is outwith the remit of this text.

MANAGEMENT

Non-surgical treatment

- Treatment is aimed at the underlying disorder, if this is known and considered treatable, although this is often unsuccessful
- Occasionally drugs (e.g. gabapentin) may be useful
- Prisms may be helpful in some instances to reduce or increase convergence
- The movement of the eyes may be reduced by giving botulinum toxin into the retrobulbar space of one eye in order to induce paralysis of all of the extraocular muscles to reduce the movement of the eye
  - The toxin is administered into the retrobulbar space using a retrobulbar needle, in a dose of 10 international units (see Chapter 15)
  - The eye takes up a neutral position in the orbit and therefore the other eye has to be closed or patched, as it will continue to move and induce double vision
  - There will be an induced ptosis due to the spread of the toxin and a ptosis prop may become a necessity
  - Botulinum toxin does not always improve the situation

Further reading

Abadi RV. Visual performances with contact lenses and congenital idiopathic nystamus. *Br J Physiol Optics* 1979; **33**: 32–7

Abadi RV, Dickinson CM. Waveform characteristics in congenital nystagmus. *Doc Ophthalmol* 1986; **64**: 153

D'Esposito M, Reccia R, Roberti G, Russo P. Amount of surgery in congenital nystagmus. *Ophthalmologica* 1989; **198**: 145–51

Fells P, Dulley B. Surgical management of compensatory head posture. *Trans Ophthalmol Soc UK* 1976; **96**: 90–5

Kestenbaum A. *Clinical methods of neuro-ophthalmic examination*, 2nd edn. Grune & Stratton, New York. 1961

Lee JP. Surgical treatment of nystagmus. *Eye* 1988; **2**: 44–7

Nelson LB, Ervin-Mulvey LD, Calhoun JH *et al.* Surgical management for abnormal head position in nystagmus: the augmented modified Kestenbaum procedure. *Br J Ophthalmol* 1984; **68**: 796–800

Pierse D. Operation on the vertical muscles in cases of nystagmus. *Br J Ophthalmol* 1959; **43**: 230–3

Pratt-Johnston JA. Complicated strabismus and adjustable sutures. *Aust NZ J Ophthalmol* 1988; **16**: 87

Ruben ST, Lee JP, O'Neil D, Dunlop I, Elston JS. The use of botulinum toxin for treatment of acquired nystagmus and oscillopsia. *Ophthalmology* 1994; **101**: 783–7

von Noorden GK, Sprunger DT. Large rectus muscle recessions for the treatment of congenital nystagmus. *Arch Ophthalmol* 1991; **109**: 221–4

PART 3
How to do it

12

Surgery on the rectus muscles

This chapter examines surgery to the rectus muscles:

Recession

Resection

Advancement

Elevation and depression of horizontal recti

Graded repositioning

Faden operation

Transposition procedures

Stay sutures

Amounts of surgery

Surgery to the horizontal rectus muscles, in the form of recessing and resecting the muscles, is commonly performed for esotropia and exotropia. These muscles can also be moved away from their original line of action to treat vertical deviations, pattern strabismus (A and V patterns) and nerve palsies. Surgery to the vertical rectus muscles is less commonly performed, but is fundamentally similar to horizontal rectus muscle surgery.

Each patient requires an individual surgical approach to the management of their squint, but the tables in Chapters 5 and 6 (reproduced in the Appendix) may be of assistance as a guide in deciding on measurements, particularly for those beginning strabismus surgery.

Standard horizontal rectus recession

Principles: The rectus muscle is detached from the globe and replaced further from the limbus. This shortens the distance between the origin and insertion of the muscle and therefore has a weakening effect.

Indications: Standard procedure for weakening a medial rectus in esotropia or lateral rectus in exotropia (usually as a bilateral procedure or combined with resection of the ipsilateral antagonist).

Method

1. Drape the eye, insert the speculum and instill adrenaline 0.01% or phenylephrine 2.5% drops to constrict the conjunctival vessels and so reduce bleeding. Place two traction sutures through the conjunctiva and episclera at the 12 and 6 o'clock positions at the limbus.

2. Make a conjunctival peritomy around the limbus in the region of the muscle for about 110°. From the edge of this make a radial incision into the conjunctiva – superomedially for the medial rectus muscle and superolaterally for the lateral rectus. Avoid the interpalpebral conjunctiva when making the radial incision (Figure 12.1a).

3. Dissect down the subconjunctival space on either side of the muscle using Westcott scissors in a spreading (not cutting) fashion. Do not dissect directly over the muscle as this tends to bleed.

4. Pass a squint hook into this area and hook the muscle (when hooking the lateral rectus this is better done from above as the inferior oblique can become caught up if hooked from below).

5. Clean the Tenon's capsule from the muscle, using blunt dissection, if possible.

6. Replace the squint hook with a Chavasse hook, which spreads the muscle.

7. Insert a 6/0 absorbable suture into each outer third of the muscle at its insertion, by passing two throws of the suture –1 full thickness and 1 partial thickness (Figure 12.1b).

8. Disinsert the muscle from the sclera using Westcott scissors, carefully preserving the suture (Figure 12.1c).

9. Measure the distance that the muscle has to be recessed using calipers (measure from limbus or previous insertion depending on preference).

10. Place the suture through the sclera (partial thickness) (Figure 12.1d), so that the tip of the needle can be seen at all times. This involves a wrist-based action.

11. When tying the suture hold the end of the suture with the needle on it and keep this taut. Run the other end of the suture down this taut end. This prevents snagging of the knot and holds the eye in the optimum position to prevent adhesion of the Tenon's capsule and the conjunctiva (Figure 12.1e).

12. The conjunctiva is closed using buried 8/0 absorbable sutures (Figure 12.1f) and an injection of local anaesthetic is given subconjunctivally over the muscle.

(a)

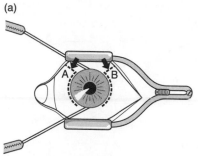

Conjunctival incisions for rectus muscle surgery

A = Approach to medial rectus with relieving incision radially and 110° limbal peritomy

B = Same for lateral rectus

Arrows mark positions for closure of the incision with sutures. Note traction sutures

(b)

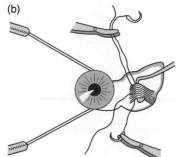

Suturing to a rectus muscle: The Chevasse squint hook lifts the muscle away from the globe. Two passes of the suture are made through the peripheral 1/3 rds of the muscle width

(c)

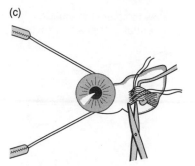

Removing the rectus muscle from the globe taking care not to cut the sutures in the process.

(d) Callipers measuring distance

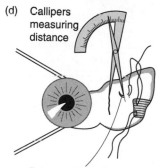

Suture pushing through partial thickness sclera

(e)

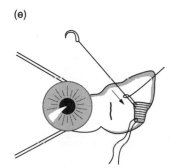

Hold end of suture with needle attached taut and run the other end down this

(f)

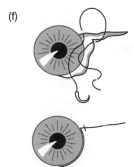

Closing the conjunctival wound: The absorbable 8/0 suture is passed from below upwards through the conjunctival edges so that the knot lies buried beneath the closed conjunctiva

Figure 12.1 Horizontal rectus muscle recession

Hang back recession

Principles: To weaken a muscle by recession, but leave the muscle hanging back from sutures attached to the original insertion rather than placing the sutures posteriorly on the globe.

How to suture the muscle
– central $\frac{1}{3}$ 2 bites and knotted

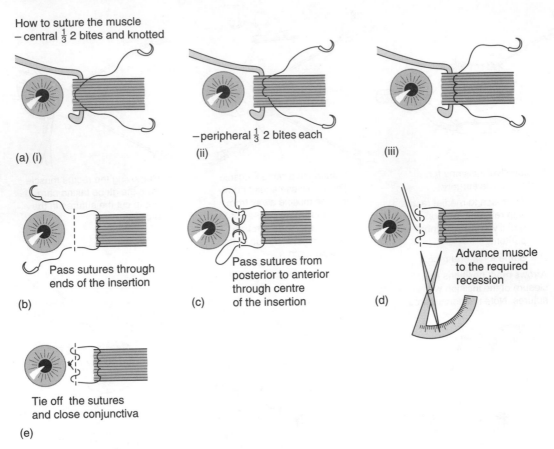

–peripheral $\frac{1}{3}$ 2 bites each

(a) (i)   (ii)   (iii)

Pass sutures through
ends of the insertion

(b)

Pass sutures from
posterior to anterior
through centre
(c)   of the insertion

Advance muscle
to the required
recession

(d)

Tie off the sutures
and close conjunctiva

(e)

Figure 12.2   Hang back recession

Indications: To weaken a rectus muscle, particularly in cases with:

- Difficult access (e.g. small baby or a very large recession required)
- High risk of perforation during suturing (e.g. very thin sclera or inexperienced surgeon)
- The use of adjustable sutures (see Chapter 14).

Also useful for the superior rectus (because of the presence of the superior oblique), and the inferior rectus (because of attachments of inferior oblique).

Method

1.   Locate and hook the rectus muscle as described above (Standard horizontal rectus recession 1–6).

2. Place a double-ended 6/0 absorbable suture through the centre third of the muscle belly just behind the insertion, taking a double bite and then lock this suture with one throw. Take a double-bite of each of the outer thirds of the muscle, each with one of the two ends (Figure 12.2a).

3. Disinsert the muscle from the sclera using Westcott scissors, carefully preserving the suture.

4. Place the two ends of the suture through the insertion with a double bite (Figure 12.2b, c). When suturing to the insertion, bites should always be from posterior to anterior, since the sclera is thin behind the insertion but thick in front. This reduces the risk of perforation.

5. Pull up or let back the muscle the required distance, measuring the distance with calipers (Figure 12.2d).

6. Tie off the suture, leaving the muscle hanging back from the original insertion (Figure 12.2e).

7. The suture is passed through a small nick of episclera in the region of the muscle end to prevent slippage (routinely by some surgeons and only for high risk cases by others).

8. Close the conjunctiva with buried 8/0 absorbable sutures and give some subconjunctival local anaesthetic.

Inferior rectus recession

Principles: Attention has to be paid to several specific points when recessing the inferior rectus. In particular, the patient must be warned that recession of the inferior rectus may cause postoperative lower lid retraction. Standard recession or hang back recession may be used but, owing to the risk of late overcorrection, adjustable sutures should be used wherever possible.

Indications:
- Hypotropia, commonly due to thyroid eye disease
- Contralateral IV nerve palsy
- Blow out fracture.

Method

1. Drape the eye, insert the speculum and instill adrenaline 0.01% or phenylephrine 2.5% drops to constrict the conjunctival vessels and so reduce bleeding. Place a traction suture at the 6 o'clock position.

2. Make an inferior 90° limbal peritomy with two relieving incisions extending inferonasally and inferotemporally (Figure 12.3a).

3. Dissect down the subconjunctival space on either side of the muscle using Westcott scissors in a spreading (not cutting) fashion. Do not dissect directly over the muscle as this tends to bleed.

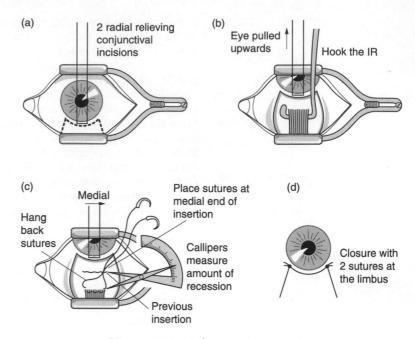

Figure 12.3 Inferior rectus recession

4. Hook the muscle under direct vision, clean the Tenon's capsule from the sides of the muscle using blunt dissection and, using sharp dissection, clear away the attachments of the lower lid retractors.

5. Replace the round-ended squint hook with a Chavasse hook which spreads the muscle (Figure 12.3b).

6. Place 6/0 absorbable sutures through the muscle as for a standard recession or as for a hang back recession, if this is preferred (see above).

7. Disinsert the muscle from the sclera using Westcott scissors, carefully preserving the suture.

8. Suture the muscle as described above, but sagittalize the muscle as this is done – i.e. move the inferior rectus medially half a muscle width (Figure 12.3c). This manoeuvre reduces the risk of a post-operative A-pattern.

9. Close the conjunctiva with buried 8/0 absorbable sutures (Figure 12.3d) and inject local anaesthetic subconjunctivally over the area of the muscle.

Superior rectus recession

Principles: The superior rectus has the tendon of the superior oblique lying between it and the sclera and so a hang back recession is recommended.

Indications:

- Hypertropia due to ipsilateral inferior rectus weakness.
- Hypertropia due to superior rectus restriction (e.g. thyroid eye disease).

Method

1. Drape the eye, insert the speculum and instill adrenaline 0.01% or phenylephrine 2.5% drops to constrict the conjunctival vessels and so reduce bleeding. Place a traction suture at the 12 o'clock position.
2. Use this to pull the eye into downgaze. Make a superior 90° limbal peritomy with two relieving incisions extending superonasally and superotemporally (Figure 12.4a).
3. Dissect down the subconjunctival space on either side of the muscle using Westcott scissors in a spreading (not cutting) fashion. Do not dissect directly over the muscle as this tends to bleed.

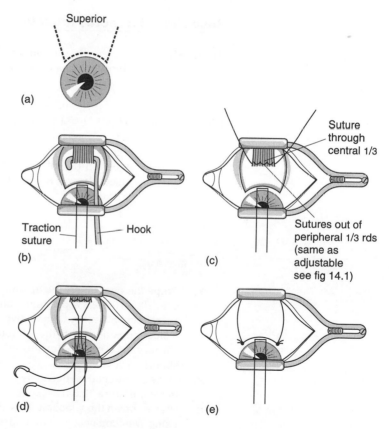

Figure 12.4 Recession of superior rectus

4. Hook the muscle under direct vision (Figure 12.4b), clean the Tenon's capsule from the sides of the muscle using blunt dissection.
5. Replace the round-ended squint hook with a Chavasse hook which spreads the muscle.
6. Place a double-ended 6/0 absorbable suture through the centre third of the muscle belly just behind the insertion. Take a double bite and then tie this suture. Take a double bite of each of the outer thirds of the muscle, one with each end of the suture (Figure 12.4c).
7. Detach the muscle from the globe, carefully preserving the suture.
8. Place each of the ends of the suture through the central third of the insertion, pointing the ends slightly towards each other (Figure 12.4d). When suturing to the insertion, bites should always be from posterior to anterior, as the sclera is thin behind the insertion but thicker in front. This reduces the risk of scleral perforation.
9. Pull up or let back the muscle the required distance.
10. Tie off the suture, close the conjunctiva with 8/0 absorbable sutures (Figure 12.4e) and give subconjunctival local anaesthetic.

Resection of a rectus muscle

Principles: A length of muscle is excised, so tightening and therefore strengthening a rectus muscle.

Indications: This is used to strengthen a muscle's actions – e.g. the lateral rectus for esotropia, the medial rectus for exotropia. It is commonly used in association with weakening of the ipsilateral antagonist. This is not used, however, in restrictive strabismus, e.g. thyroid eye disease.

Method

1. Drape the eye, insert the speculum and instill adrenaline 0.01% or phenylephrine 2.5% drops to constrict the conjunctival vessels and so reduce bleeding. Place two 6/0 traction sutures at 6 and 12 o'clock positions at the limbus for horizontal rectus muscle surgery, at 6 o'clock for the inferior rectus and 12 o'clock for the superior rectus.
2. Make a conjunctival peritomy and radial incision in the region of the muscle (Figure 12.5a).
3. Dissect down the subconjunctival space on either side of the muscle using Westcott scissors in a spreading (not cutting) fashion. Do not dissect directly over the muscle as this tends to bleed.

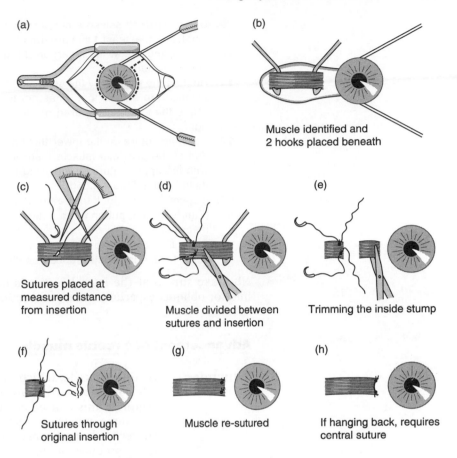

(a)

(b)

Muscle identified and
2 hooks placed beneath

(c)

Sutures placed at
measured distance
from insertion

(d)

Muscle divided between
sutures and insertion

(e)

Trimming the inside stump

(f)

Sutures through
original insertion

(g)

Muscle re-sutured

(h)

If hanging back, requires
central suture

Figure 12.5   Rectus muscle resection

4.   Pass a squint hook into this area and hook the muscle (when hooking the lateral rectus this is better done from above as the inferior oblique can become caught up if hooked from below).

5.   Clean the Tenon's capsule from the muscle, using blunt dissection, if possible.

6.   Replace the round hook with a Chavasse squint hook and spread the muscle between the 2 squint hooks, placing the Chavasse at the area down the muscle that is going to require suturing (Figure 12.5b).

7.   Measure the length of the muscle to be resected using calipers. Place the 6/0 absorbable sutures through each outer third of the muscle at this measure (Figure 12.5c). One suture is full thickness, the other partial thickness.

8.   Apply straight artery forceps across the muscle, proximal to the sutures and gently crush the muscle. Apply gentle diathermy across the crushed area.

9. Using Westcott scissors cut across the muscle at this site, taking small bites, at least 1 mm proximal to the sutures (Figure 12.5d).
10. Cut the muscle at the insertion (Figure 12.5e) – further diathermy may be required.
11. Holding the muscle by the sutures, pull it towards the insertion and inspect it to ensure that it has not twisted. It may be necessary to rotate the eye into the area of the muscle, especially if it is quite tight.
12. Pass the suture on the lower third of the muscle through the lower end of the previous muscle insertion (Figure 12.5f). Do the same with the upper suture so ensuring that the muscle is spread out to its full width (Figure 12.5g).
13. Inspect the muscle. If the centre is hanging back from the insertion (Figure 12.5h), put an extra suture through this and tie it up to the insertion.
14. Close the conjunctiva with buried 8/0 absorbable sutures and inject some local anaesthetic subconjunctivally.

NB Make sure that the lateral rectus is freed from attachments to the inferior oblique, especially in large resections and re-operations.

Advancement of a rectus muscle

Principles: A rectus muscle, which has previously been recessed, is advanced forwards towards its original insertion. If required, this can be combined with resecting some of the same muscle. When calculating the amount of surgery to be performed, allow for the fact that advancement produces a slightly greater effect than resection. Ideally such surgery should be carried out using adjustable sutures as the result tends to be unpredictable.

Indications:

- To the medial rectus – consecutive exotropia following esotropia surgery (usually combined with lateral rectus recession).
- To the inferior rectus – overcorrection following inferior rectus recession.
- To the lateral rectus – consecutive esotropia following exotropia surgery (less common).
- To the superior rectus – overcorrection following superior rectus surgery.

Method

1. Locate and hook the muscle as described above (Resection of a rectus muscle 1–5), bearing in mind the muscle is in a recessed position and may have scar tissue around it due to previous surgery.

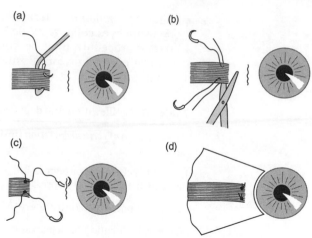

Figure 12.6   Advancement of a rectus muscle

2.   Place a Chavasse hook beneath the muscle (Figure 12.6a).
3.   Take two bites of each outer third of the muscle, one partial thickness and one full thickness (Figure 12.6a) using 2 single ended 6/0 absorbable sutures. If some resection is to be performed, place these sutures a measured distance behind the point of attachment of the rectus muscle to the eye.
4.   Using Westcott scissors, cut across the muscle, just proximal to the sutures, taking small bites (Figure 12.6b). Diathermy may be required.
5.   Holding the muscle by the sutures, pull it towards its previous insertion to ensure that it has not twisted. It may be necessary to rotate the eye into the area of the muscle, especially if it is quite tight.
6.   Pass the suture on the lower third of the muscle through the lower end of the original muscle insertion. Do the same with the upper suture so ensuring that the muscle is spread out to its full width (Figure 12.6c and d).
7.   Close the conjunctiva with buried 8/0 absorbable sutures and inject some local anaesthetic subconjunctivally.

If using adjustables see Chapter 14.

Elevation or depression of the insertion of the medial and lateral rectus muscles

Principles:

- The horizontal rectus muscles are re-sutured to the globe higher or lower than the original insertion. This introduces a small vertical element when the muscles of the same eye are moved in the same direction (Table 12.1).

- Bilateral medial or lateral rectus movement in the same direction of opposite eyes collapses V or A patterns (Table 12.1).
- Either procedure may be combined with a recession/resection procedure of the horizontal muscles to treat any associated horizontal deviation.

Table 12.1 Elevation and depression of the horizontal rectus muscles

For correction of vertical deviation (ipsilateral MR and LR moved in the same direction):

Half width elevation or depression	5–10 dioptres of height corrected
Full width elevation or depression	10–15 dioptres of height corrected

For A or V patterns (contralateral MRs or LRs moved in the same direction):

Half width elevation or depression	collapse pattern by 10 dioptres
Full width elevation or depression	collapse pattern by up to 20 dioptres

- Place the medial rectus muscles towards the apex of a pattern i.e. downwards in a V pattern and upwards in an A pattern and vice versa for the lateral rectus (Figure 12.7a, b)
- These procedures can be combined with a resection or recession of the rectus muscle
- Expect relatively more effect in larger deviations

Indications:

- To correct small vertical deviations (<15 dioptres) in conjunction with horizontal squints (e.g. third nerve palsies to improve cosmesis or concomitant squints with a vertical element).
  - For correction of vertical deviation the ipsilateral MR and LR are moved in the same direction. Upwards to improve elevation and downwards to lower the eye.
- To correct an A or V pattern
  - Move the MRs towards apex of pattern (Figures 7.2 and 7.4), i.e. downwards in a V pattern and upwards in an A pattern
  - Move the LRs in the opposite direction away from the apex (Figures 7.2 and 7.4)
  - For A and V patterns this procedure is good when performing bilateral surgery (e.g. bilateral medial rectus recessions) but when a recess/resect procedure is used on one eye only, it may be better to perform graded weakening to avoid unwanted torsion (see below and Figures 7.3 and 7.5).

Method

1. Expose the rectus muscle for resection or recession in the usual way (see above) and detach the muscle from the globe.
2. To elevate the muscle one half width, take the lower of the two sutures and reattach it to the eye in line with the centre of the insertion (Figure 12.7a (i, ii)).

3. For a full width elevation place the suture through the top of the insertion. Place the other suture one full insertion width higher.

4. To depress the muscle one half width, take the upper of the two sutures and reattach it to the eye in line with the centre of the insertion.

5. For a full width depression, place the suture through the bottom of the insertion. Place the other suture one full insertion width lower (Figure 12.7b(i, ii)).

6. Ensure that the new insertion line lies parallel to the original insertion line.

7. Close the conjunctiva with buried 8/0 absorbable sutures and inject local anaesthetic subconjunctivally.

(i) Elevation of horizontal rectus $\frac{1}{2}$ muscle width

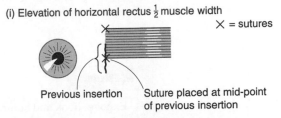

$\times$ = sutures

Previous insertion   Suture placed at mid-point of previous insertion

(ii) Depression of horizontal rectus $\frac{1}{2}$ muscle width

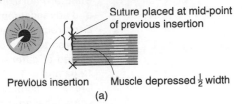

Suture placed at mid-point of previous insertion

Previous insertion   Muscle depressed $\frac{1}{2}$ width

(a)

(i) Depression muscle insertion-full muscle width

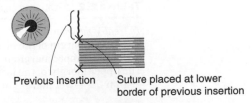

Previous insertion   Suture placed at lower border of previous insertion

(ii) Elevation of muscle insertion-full muscle width

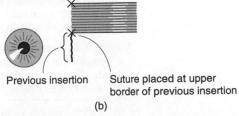

Previous insertion   Suture placed at upper border of previous insertion

(b)

Figure 12.7   Depression of horizontal recti

Graded replacement of the horizontal rectus muscles

Principles: The upper and lower parts of the medial or lateral rectus muscles are re-sutured to the globe at different distances from the limbus (or previous insertion) to correct A or V patterns (Table 2.2).

Indications: A or V patterns not associated with oblique overaction or underaction. This is particularly useful when doing recess/resect surgery to one eye only, since elevating and depressing the insertions of two rectus muscles on the same eye may lead to unwanted torsional effects (Figures 7.3 and 7.5).

Method

1. Expose, hook and suture the muscle as for a recession, resection or advancement procedure via a limbal conjunctival incision. (see Standard horizontal rectus recession, resection of a rectus muscle and advancement of a rectus muscle above).
2. Each rectus muscle is recessed or resected as required and is re-sutured to the globe, but the superior suture and inferior suture are placed at different distances from the limbus (Figures 7.3, 7.5 and 12.8a and b, Table 12.2)
3. Close the conjunctiva with buried 8/0 absorbable sutures and inject some local anaesthetic subconjunctivally.

Table 12.2 Graded recession/resection of the horizontal rectus muscles

---

To treat V patterns
The lower margin of the medial rectus is placed in a preferentially weaker position than the upper margin in a V pattern
The upper margin of the lateral rectus is placed in a preferentially weaker position than the lower margin in a V pattern

To treat A patterns
The upper margin of the medial rectus is placed in a preferentially weaker position than the lower margin in an A pattern
The lower margin of the lateral rectus is placed in a preferentially weaker position than the upper margin in an A pattern

A 2 mm difference between the upper and lower borders of the muscle closes up to 15 dioptres of A or V pattern
A 3 mm difference between the upper and lower borders of the muscle closes up to 20–25 dioptres of A or V pattern

---

- Either procedure can be combined with a recession or a resection of the horizontal muscle

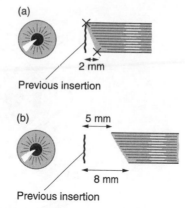

Figure 12.8   Selective replacement of horizontal recti

Faden operation

Principles: A non-absorbable suture is placed through the belly of the muscle and the sclera in the region of the equator of the eye. This tethers the muscle to the globe. This operation has little or no effect on the deviation in the primary position, but weakens the muscle progressively as it moves into its direction of action. It is used in cases with rectus muscle overaction but no deviation in the primary position.

Indications:

- Convergence excess esotropia (medial recti).
- Blow out fracture of the orbit with diplopia on downgaze despite good depression (contralateral inferior rectus).
- Recovered VI nerve palsy with persistent diplopia on abduction (contralateral medial rectus).
- Diplopia on contralateral gaze following surgery for exotropia (contralateral medial rectus).

Relative contraindications:

- The Faden procedure is not very effective when used on the lateral rectus, because of the long arc of contact that this muscle has with the globe.
- It can be difficult to perform on the superior rectus since this muscle is already inserted rather posteriorly, the fibres of the superior oblique lie below it and a vortex vein sits at the region that a suture would be placed.
- A Faden of the superior rectus is probably not sufficient to deal with dissociated vertical divergence in the long term.

(a)

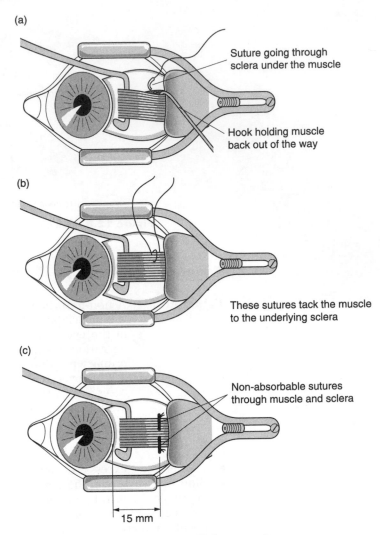

Suture going through
sclera under the muscle

Hook holding muscle
back out of the way

(b)

These sutures tack the muscle
to the underlying sclera

(c)

Non-absorbable sutures
through muscle and sclera

15 mm

Figure 12.9 Faden operation

Method

1. Locate and hook the muscle as described above (Resection of a rectus muscle 1– 6).
2. Insert a retractor (e.g. Fison retractor) to hold the conjunctiva away from the muscles to enable exposure of the rectus muscle right back behind the equator. Identify the locations of the emissary vortex veins and carefully preserve them.
3. Using a 5/0 non-absorbable braided suture take a partial thickness bite through the sclera underneath the border of the muscle. This should be about 15 mm from the limbus (Figure 12.9a). The sclera

is thick here (c.1 mm) but extra care should be taken not to perforate the eye since any damage to the retina in such a posterior position would produce visual symptoms.

4. Continue the bite with the suture to take in one third of the muscle width in a double throw and tie the suture, so that the suture tacks the muscle firmly to the underlying sclera (Figure 12.9b).

5. Perform the same procedure with the other side of the muscle belly so that there are two sutures locating the edges of the muscle belly to the sclera at this point (Figure 12.9c). If access is very awkward it may be easier to leave the first suture untied, on a bulldog clip, until the second suture is ready to tie.

6. Close the conjunctiva and give subconjunctival local anaesthesia as for normal recess/resect procedures.

Postoperatively a Faden procedure can be a little more uncomfortable than average strabismus surgery and the patient should be warned about this and postoperative analgesia given accordingly.

Transposition surgery

Principles: Two rectus muscles are transposed away from their usual anatomical position to allow them to take up some of the action of a weakened or palsied muscle.

Indications:

- Abduction defect, e.g. total VI nerve palsy (vertical recti transposed temporally – in combination with toxin – see below).
- Depression defect, e.g. inferior rectus palsy (horizontal recti transposed downwards).
- Elevation defect, e.g. elevator palsy (horizontal recti transposed upwards).
- Adduction defect (vertical recti transposed medially and also resected 5 mm in order to provide an adequate adducting effect).

Contraindications:

- Care should be made when transposing the recti muscles because several anterior ciliary arteries are being transected. At least three months should be allowed between previous squint surgery and a transposition procedure to allow the posterior ciliary arteries to hypertrophy.
- Ensure that there is no restriction to movement (forced duction test), this operation is only useful for cases of weakness.
- This procedure is not very effective in replacing the function of the medial rectus. In this case at least a 5 mm resection of the transposing muscles should also be performed.

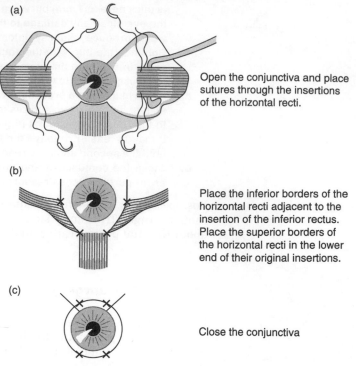

(a) Open the conjunctiva and place sutures through the insertions of the horizontal recti.

(b) Place the inferior borders of the horizontal recti adjacent to the insertion of the inferior rectus. Place the superior borders of the horizontal recti in the lower end of their original insertions.

(c) Close the conjunctiva

Figure 12.10   Full muscle transposition

- In VI nerve palsies, this procedure will not be effective if the ipsilateral MR is not weakened and this should be done prior to the surgery using botulinum toxin.

Method

1. Insert stay sutures at the 6 and 12 o'clock positions.
2. Make two radial relieving incisions on each side of the muscle to be strengthened and perform generous limbal peritomies so as to gain access to the adjacent rectus muscles.
3. Dissect out and hook each muscle to be transposed in turn and attach sutures to the insertion as in a recession (Standard horizontal rectus recession 3–8) (Figure 12.10a).
4. Move each muscle towards the weakened or palsied muscle that is to be strengthened. Suture the edge of the muscle proximal to the palsied muscle to the outer border of the insertion of the palsied muscle (Figure 12.10b).
5. Suture the distal side to the outer insertion of the moved muscle (Figure 12.10b).
6. Close the conjunctiva with buried 8/0 absorbable sutures (Figure 12.10c) and inject subconjunctival local anaesthetic.

Potential postoperative problems:

- Anterior segment ischaemia
- Development of a secondary deviation. This is most common with transposition of the vertical recti, when an unwanted vertical squint may develop. This can be managed with botulinum toxin or with a second operation to recess/resect the transposed muscles.
- Poor globe movement due to scarring – especially in cases who have had a lot of surgery.

Toxin transposition

Principles: The medial rectus is weakened by injection of botulinum toxin and a full transposition of the superior and inferior recti laterally is carried out to replace the function of the palsied lateral rectus. The anterior ciliary arteries of the lateral and medial recti are preserved, thereby reducing the risk of anterior segment ischaemia.

Indication: Totally unrecovered lateral rectus palsy.

Method

1. Inject the ipsilateral medial rectus with botulinum toxin approximately one week prior to the surgery (Figure 12.11a). If there has been little effect, it is possible to repeat the injection on the day of surgery at the end of the transposition.
2. Make two radial relieving incisions above and below the lateral rectus and perform generous limbal peritomies so as to gain access to the superior and inferior recti (Figure 12.11b). Hook the inferior rectus, place sutures in it and detach it from the globe, as one would for an inferior rectus recession.
3. Hook the lateral rectus. This still has a covering of conjunctiva, but do not diathermy the anterior ciliary artery of the lateral rectus.
4. Suture the lateral border of the inferior rectus to the inferior border of the lateral rectus at its insertion (Figure 12.11c).
5. Suture the medial border of the inferior rectus to its previous lateral insertion (Figure 12.11c).
6. Repeat this for the superior rectus, taking care not to disrupt the sutures of the inferior rectus when hooking the lateral rectus (Figure 12.11d).
7. Close the conjunctiva with buried 8/0 absorbable sutures and inject subconjunctival local anaesthetic.
8. An ideal result is for the eye to be in an exotropic position following this procedure, which will reduce as the botulinum toxin wears off.

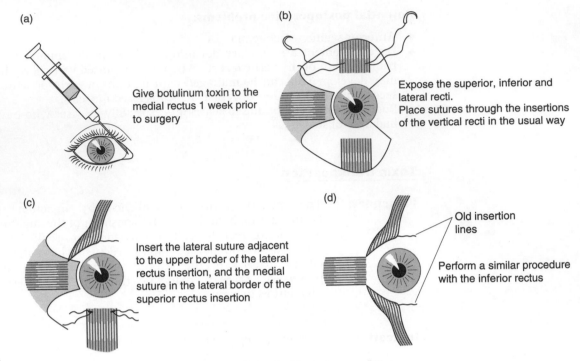

(a) Give botulinum toxin to the medial rectus 1 week prior to surgery

(b) Expose the superior, inferior and lateral recti.
Place sutures through the insertions of the vertical recti in the usual way

(c) Insert the lateral suture adjacent to the upper border of the lateral rectus insertion, and the medial suture in the lateral border of the superior rectus insertion

(d) Old insertion lines
Perform a similar procedure with the inferior rectus

Figure 12.11 Toxin transposition

Complications:

- Residual esotropia after the botulinum toxin has worn off. If this occurs, recess either one or both medial recti after three months.
- Persistent exotropia, with reduced adduction even after the toxin has worn off.
- Secondary vertical deviations.
- Anterior segment ischaemia.

Partial-width transposition procedures

The Jensen and Hummelsheim procedures were developed to provide abduction of the eye in cases of VI nerve palsy, before the advent of botulinum toxin, as they do not interfere with the blood supply of the anterior segment as much as complete transpositions. They may still be useful in areas of the world where toxin is not available but they are not as predictable and carry more risk than toxin transposition surgery and therefore are not recommended.

The Hummelsheim procedure, in which only the temporal halves of the rectus muscles are transposed, and combined with a recession of the medial rectus, is not recommended as the results are poor and re operations are often necessary.

The Jensen procedure involves splitting the bellies of the superior and inferior rectus muscles along their length and attaching them to the belly of the lateral rectus muscle – which has also been split lengthwise – to produce some abduction. The medial rectus is recessed at the same time.

Stay sutures (traction sutures)

Principles: Stay sutures are placed through the insertion of one or more rectus muscles to hold the eye in a certain position following extraocular muscle surgery.

Indications: To hold the eye in position following strabismus surgery – usually when orbital or muscular forces are not favourable to this position (e.g. in total III nerve palsies to hold the eye in adduction and slight elevation).

> **Method**

This example is for a III nerve palsy, but the position can be altered depending on the diagnosis and therefore the optimum position for the eye.

1. Place a 6/0 double ended non-absorbable suture through the insertion of the superior rectus and another through the insertion of the inferior rectus muscle, following surgical correction of the strabismus (Figure 12.12a). This is usually done transconjunctivally.

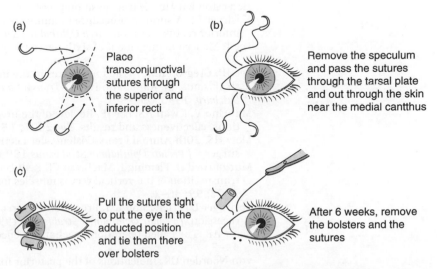

(a) Place transconjunctival sutures through the superior and inferior recti

(b) Remove the speculum and pass the sutures through the tarsal plate and out through the skin near the medial cantthus

(c) Pull the sutures tight to put the eye in the adducted position and tie them there over bolsters

After 6 weeks, remove the bolsters and the sutures

Figure 12.12 Traction sutures for III nerve palsy

2. Remove the speculum and pass each end of each suture through the medial end of the tarsal plate and out through the skin near the medial canthus as far medially as possible in order to hold the eye in a fully adducted position (Figure 12.12b) and tie over bolsters (Figure 12.12c).

3. Leave in position for up to 6 weeks (or as long as the patient can tolerate the sutures until the 6 weeks is up).

The eye remains partially closed in the postoperative period and the lids tend to be quite swollen.

Further reading

Burke JP, Keech RV. Effectiveness of inferior transposition of the horizontal rectus muscles for acquired inferior rectus paresis. *J Pediatr Ophthalmol Strabismus* 1995; **32**: 172–7

Capo H, Repka MX, Guyton DL. Hang-back lateral rectus recessions for exotropia. *J Pediatr Ophthalmol Strabismus* 1989; **26**: 31

Fells P. Vertical rectus muscle transplantation to restore abduction. In: Mein J, Bierlaagh JJM, Brummelkamp-Dons TE (eds). *Orthoptics, Transactions of the Second International Orthoptic Congress, Amsterdam*, 1972; 229–37

Fells P, Marsh RJ. Anterior segment ischemia following surgery on two rectus muscles. In: Reinecke RD (ed.) *Strabismus.* Grune & Stratton, New York. 1978; 375–80

Fitzsimmons R, Lee JP, Elston J. Treatment of sixth nerve palsy in adults with combined botulinum toxin chemodenervation and surgery. *Ophthalmology* 1998; **95**: 1535–42

deB Ribeiro G, Brooks SE, Archer SM, Del monte MA. Vertical shift of the medial rectus muscles in the treatment of A-pattern esotropia: analysis of outcome. *J Pediatr Ophthalmol Strabismus* 1995; **32**: 167–71

Helveston EM Muscle transposition procedures. *Surv Ophthalmol* 1997; **16**: 92–7

Kushner BJ. A surgical procedure to minimize lower eyelid retraction with inferior rectus recession. *Arch Ophthalmol* 1992; **110**: 1011

Lee J. Modern management of sixth nerve palsy. *Aust NZJ Ophthalmol* 1992; **20**: 41–6

Lee JP, Gregson RMC. Traction sutures in the management of fixed divergent strabismus. In: Kaufmann H (ed.) *Transactions of the 21st ESA Meeting, Salzburg*, 1993; 397–9

Maurino V, Kwan AS, Lee JP. Review of the inverse Knapp procedure: indications, effectiveness and results. *Eye* 2001; **15**: 7–11

Metz HS. 20th Annual Frank Costenbader Lecture – Muscle transposition surgery. *J Pediatr Ophthalmol Strabismus* 1993; **30**: 346–53

Murgatroyd H, Fleming I, MacEwen CJ. Reduced adduction following lateral transposition of the vertical rectus muscles for sixth nerve palsy. *Br Orthoptic J* 2002; **59**: 30–2.

Sprunger DT, Helveston EM. Progressive overcorrection after inferior rectus recession. *J Pediatr Ophthalmol Strabismus* 1993; **30**: 145–8

Scott AB. The Faden operation: mechanical effects. *Am Orthoptic J* 1977; **27**: 44–7

von Noorden GK. Indications of the posterior fixation operation in strabismus. *Ophthalmology* 1978; **85**: 512

13

Oblique muscle surgery

This chapter covers:

Inferior oblique muscle surgery
- Disinsertion
- Recession
- Anteriorization

Superior oblique surgery
- Tuck
- Posterior tenotomy
- Free tenotomy
- Harado-Ito

Surgery to the oblique muscles is more complex than surgery to the recti. This is because surgical location and identification of these muscles is more difficult. This chapter looks at methods of weakening and strengthening the inferior and superior oblique muscles.

Inferior oblique disinsertion

Principles: The inferior oblique is freed from the globe and allowed to re-attach itself at a recessed location on the globe.

Indications: Inferior oblique overaction (primary or secondary).

Method

1. Drape the eye and instill adrenaline 0.01% or phenylephrine 2.5% drops to constrict the conjunctival vessels and so reduce bleeding. Place a 6/0 silk traction suture through the inferotemporal conjunctiva and episclera and use this to hold the eye in elevation and adduction (Figure 13.1a).
2. Make a 1 cm conjunctival incision in the inferotemporal fornix (Figure 13.1b). Ensure that the incision is through the Tenon's

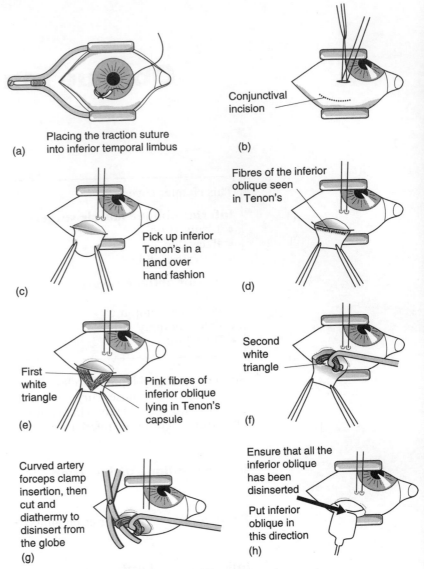

(a) Placing the traction suture into inferior temporal limbus

(b) Conjunctival incision

(c) Pick up inferior Tenon's in a hand over hand fashion

(d) Fibres of the inferior oblique seen in Tenon's

(e) First white triangle — Pink fibres of inferior oblique lying in Tenon's capsule

(f) Second white triangle

(g) Curved artery forceps clamp insertion, then cut and diathermy to disinsert from the globe

(h) Ensure that all the inferior oblique has been disinserted — Put inferior oblique in this direction

Figure 13.1 Inferior oblique disinsertion

capsule and right down onto the sclera. Lift up the conjunctiva and subconjunctival tissues on the inferior aspect of this incision and pick up these tissues, looking at the inner aspect, in a hand over hand fashion using Moorfields forceps (one pair in each hand) (Figure 13.1c). The pink fibres of the inferior oblique should be seen lying within the Tenon's capsule (Figure 13.1d).

3. Lift up these fibres until it is possible to see behind them – the first 'white triangle' (Figure 13.1e). Pass a squint hook into the apex of

this triangle, behind the pink fibres, to expose the belly of the muscle. If the squint hook does not pass through the Tenon's with ease it is likely that not all the muscle has been hooked.

4. When the muscle has been hooked it should be possible to see the sclera below and behind the muscle – the second 'white triangle' (Figure 13.1f). If the muscle has been split by the action of the squint hook, or if the inferior oblique has a bifid belly, then the sclera will not be visible and the muscle must be re-hooked.

5. Place a curved artery forceps along the muscle belly as far towards the insertion as possible and clamp the muscle as it attaches to the sclera along the lower border of the lateral rectus (Figure 13.1g). Remove the clamp and diathermy across the clamp line. Cut the muscle at this point, carefully holding onto its end. This is muscle tissue and may yet bleed, so further diathermy of this is usually required. Gently push the inferior oblique downwards and medially into the subconjunctival space.

6. Place a retractor in the conjunctival wound and examine the sclera. Make sure no muscle fibres remain attached to the globe (Figure 13.1h).

7. The conjunctiva may be sutured, but this is not necessary.

Inferior oblique recession

Principle: This procedure is identical to inferior oblique disinsertion, except that the inferior oblique is sutured to the globe rather than left free to find its own attachment to the sclera. Studies have confirmed that the two procedures are equally effective.

Indications: Re-do operations for inferior oblique overaction (primary or secondary). Some surgeons choose to use this procedure for all cases of inferior oblique overaction, but most reserve it for re-operations where the postoperative location of the inferior oblique needs to be known precisely.

Method

1. Locate and hook the inferior oblique as described above (Inferior oblique disinsertion 1–4).

2. After applying diathermy and cutting the inferior oblique at its insertion, pass a single-ended 6/0 absorbable suture through the anterior corner of the muscle (Figure 13.2a).

3. Pass a squint hook into the conjunctival wound and behind the insertion of the inferior rectus (Figure 13.2b). This should not require an extension of the conjunctival wound. Measure 3 mm

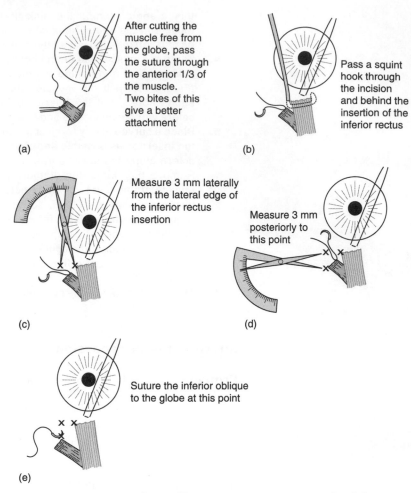

Figure 13.2 Inferior oblique recession: suturing to the globe

lateral and 3 mm posterior to the lateral margin of the insertion of this muscle (Figure 13.2c, d).

4. Anchor the inferior oblique to the globe with the 6/0 suture at this point (Figure 13.2e).

5. The conjunctiva should be sutured with an 8/0 absorbable suture as it tends to gape more than in a simple disinsertion.

Inferior oblique anteriorization

Principles: The inferior oblique is detached from the globe and is re-attached anteriorly so that it becomes a passive restrictor of upgaze.

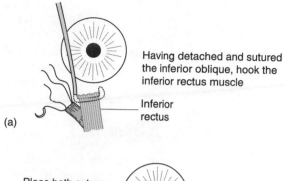

Having detached and sutured the inferior oblique, hook the inferior rectus muscle

Inferior rectus

(a)

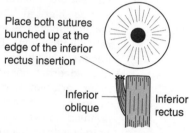

Place both sutures bunched up at the edge of the inferior rectus insertion

Inferior oblique

Inferior rectus

(b)

Figure 13.3   Inferior oblique anteriorization

Indications: Dissociated vertical divergence, especially when also occurring with inferior oblique overaction.

Method

1. Locate the inferior oblique as described above (Inferior oblique dis-insertion 1–4). Detach it from the globe and pass a 6/0 absorbable suture through both corners of the detached muscle (Figure 13.3a).
2. Pass a squint hook into the conjunctival wound and behind the inferior rectus insertion. It may be necessary to extend the conjunctival wound in order to gain a view of the insertion, but this is not usually necessary.
3. Suture both sides of the inferior oblique adjacent to the lateral aspect of the insertion of the inferior rectus in a 'bunched up' fashion (Figure 13.3b).
4. Close the conjunctiva with a buried 8/0 absorbable suture.
5. The procedure leaves a lump at the site of the inferior rectus insertion, but this fades away with time.

Superior oblique tuck

Principles: A lax superior oblique tendon is tightened to improve superior oblique function, but not over-tightened so as to produce an iatrogenic Brown's syndrome. A superior oblique tuck improves both the depressor and the torsional functions of the muscle.

Indications: Superior oblique weakness, in which the pattern of weakness is maximum in depression in adduction. This is especially useful in congenital weakness in which the superior oblique tendon may be very lax.

Method

1. Place a 6/0 traction suture though the superior limbal conjunctiva and episclera at 12 o'clock and pull the eye into downgaze. Open the conjunctiva with a superior limbal peritomy and two radial relieving incisions (Figure 13.4a).

2. Pass a squint hook under the superior rectus muscle and clean off any adherent connective tissue, while preserving the anterior ciliary arteries. Use the squint hook to pull the eye into a position of downgaze. Remove the speculum and retract the upper lid and conjunctiva with a Desmarres retractor instead. An assistant must hold both the hook and the retractor (Figure 13.4b).

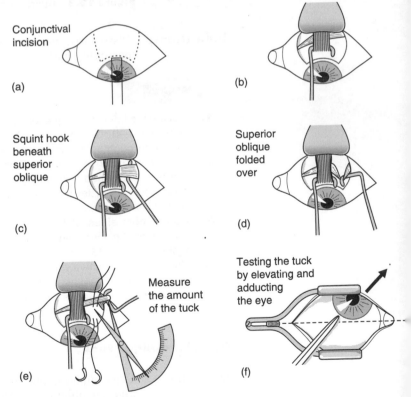

Conjunctival incision

(a)

(b)

Squint hook beneath superior oblique

(c)

Superior oblique folded over

(d)

Measure the amount of the tuck

(e)

Testing the tuck by elevating and adducting the eye

(f)

Figure 13.4 Superior oblique tuck

3. Identify the superior oblique tendon on the temporal side of the superior rectus. The fibres of the superior oblique run backwards under the belly of the superior rectus from nasal to temporal (Figure 13.4c). They are quite diaphanous in appearance and may easily be missed and considered part of the episcleral tissue. The anterior edge may be elevated using an iris repositor or a flat squint hook. Once identified pass a hook beneath them on the temporal aspect of the superior rectus. The fibres are very strong and will intort and depress the globe if gently pulled on.

4. Lift the superior oblique tendon away from the globe with a hook and pull it towards its insertion, so that it folds over (Figure 13.4d). Pass a 5/0 non-absorbable suture through the proximal tendon and into the insertion. It is better to use a coloured suture. Tie the suture with bows. Measure the amount of the tuck (twice the distance from the insertion to the squint hook under the superior oblique (Figure13.4e). A tendon tucker is available and makes this operation easier.

Note: In cases of congenital weakness of the superior oblique, the tendon can be very lax and a tuck of as much as 15 mm may be performed. In acquired cases the amount is usually much less, e.g. 6–8 mm.

5. Test the effect of this amount of surgery: remove all the squint hooks and the retractor and replace the speculum. Grasp the limbus at the 6 o'clock position with toothed forceps and elevate the eye in a position of adduction, while gently pushing the eye back towards the apex of the orbit. If the tuck is the correct amount the inferior limbus will elevate to the middle of the interpalpebral zone (Figure 13.4f) with ease and then develop a feeling of resistance. If the tuck is too great, there will be marked resistance to passive elevation prior to this level and if insufficient there will be little or no resistance.

6. If the tuck is not correct, remove the 5/0 sutures from the superior oblique and replace them so that either less or more tendon is tucked. Re-test.

7. When the tuck is correct, tie off the 5/0 sutures and cut them. The tucked tendon may lie neater if it is tacked to the globe. Close the conjunctiva with buried 8/0 absorbable sutures.

Complications:
- A small Brown's-type restriction may occur post-operatively, but this almost always vanishes after a few weeks.
- If re-operation is necessary, be grateful that you used coloured sutures.

Posterior tenotomy of the superior oblique

Principle: The posterior portion of the superior oblique is selectively weakened, so reducing the depressor action but not the torsional function of the muscle.

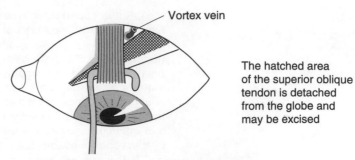

Vortex vein

The hatched area
of the superior oblique
tendon is detached
from the globe and
may be excised

Figure 13.5 Posterior tenotomy of the superior oblique

Indications:
- A-pattern exotropia with superior oblique overaction, commonly caused by:
  - primary superior oblique overaction
  - dysthyroid eye disease following inferior rectus weakening
- To balance a weak contralateral inferior rectus muscle (to reduce the overaction of depression in adduction, without affecting torsion)

Method

1. Expose the superior oblique tendon as above (Superior oblique tuck 1–3).
2. Identify the full width of the superior oblique tendon temporal to the superior rectus, ensuring that the posterior edge of it can be identified. There is a vortex vein at this point that provides a good landmark.
3. Split the tendon lengthwise, under the superior rectus muscle, dividing the anterior 20% of the tendon from the posterior 80%.
4. Disinsert the posterior 80% of the tendon from the globe, allowing it to retract freely under the superior rectus muscle and beyond (Figure 13.5).
5. Remove the retractor and squint hooks, re-insert the speculum and close the conjunctiva with buried 8/0 absorbable sutures.

Free tenotomy of the superior oblique

Principle: The superior oblique tendon is completely divided to reduce or abolish the function of the muscle.

Indications: Brown's syndrome.

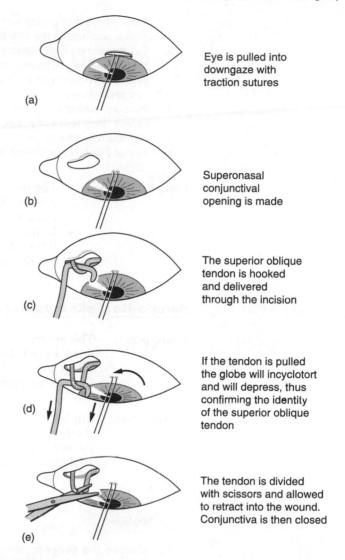

(a) Eye is pulled into downgaze with traction sutures

(b) Superonasal conjunctival opening is made

(c) The superior oblique tendon is hooked and delivered through the incision

(d) If the tendon is pulled the globe will incyclotort and will depress, thus confirming the identity of the superior oblique tendon

(e) The tendon is divided with scissors and allowed to retract into the wound. Conjunctiva is then closed

Figure 13.6 Free tenotomy of superior oblique (nasal disinsertion)

Method

1. Place a 6/0 traction suture though the superior limbal conjunctiva and episclera at 12 o'clock and pull the eye into downgaze. Perform a superonasal conjunctival incision (Figure 13.6a, b).
2. Identify the superior oblique tendon on the nasal side of the superior rectus. The fibres of the superior oblique run from the trochlea backwards under the belly of the superior rectus and the nasal fibres appear as a round cord nasal to the superior rectus. Hook

these fibres and gently pull on them; this will intort and depress the globe, confirming the identity of the tendon (Figure 13.6c, d).

3.   Cut the fibres with Westcott scissors and allow them to separate (Figure 13.6e). Ensure that the connective tissue between the superior rectus and the superior oblique is not damaged during this procedure.

4.   Passive elevation of the eye in adduction should be carried out before the tenotomy and repeated afterwards to confirm that elevation in adduction is much freer.

5.   The conjunctiva is closed using buried 8/0 absorbable sutures.

Complications:
- The Brown's pattern will persist in the immediate postoperative period, but should gradually disappear
- In the long term patients may develop symptoms from the superior oblique weakness, and may require an inferior oblique weakening procedure.

Harado-Ito (Fells modification)

Principle: The anterior fibres of the superior oblique are strengthened by advancing them to increase their ability to intort the eye. The posterior fibres are not advanced so that an iatrogenic Brown's syndrome is not produced.

Indications: Superior oblique paresis with predominantly excyclotorsion. Such patients tend to have bilateral acquired IV nerve palsies in which the vertical deviations tend to balance out. The procedure is usually performed bilaterally.

Method

1.   Expose the superior oblique tendon on the temporal side of the superior rectus muscle as above (see Superior oblique tuck 1–3).

2.   Identify the full width of the superior oblique temporal to the superior rectus. Split the tendon so that the squint hook lies only beneath the anterior 50% of the tendon (Figure 13.7a).

3.   Place two 6/0 absorbable sutures through the margins of this anterior 50% of the tendon as one would for a rectus muscle (Figure 13.7b). The fibres of the tendon are very thin, but are quite tough and suturing is possible. Detach the anterior 50% of the tendon from the globe and extend the division up the tendon to beneath the superior rectus (Figure 13.7c).

4.   Place a squint hook beneath the insertion of the lateral rectus muscle. A small increase in the conjunctival incision may be required, but this is not usual. Advance this anterior 50% of the

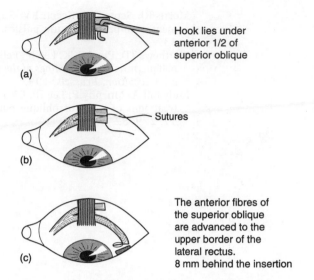

(a) Hook lies under anterior 1/2 of superior oblique

(b) Sutures

(c) The anterior fibres of the superior oblique are advanced to the upper border of the lateral rectus. 8 mm behind the insertion

Figure 13.7 Harada–Ito procedure (Fell's modification)

superior oblique tendon temporally and suture it to the globe, as close as possible to the upper aspect of the lateral rectus muscle. The anterior of the two sutures should lie approximately 8 mm behind the lateral rectus muscle insertion.

5. Close the conjunctiva with buried 8/0 absorbable sutures.

Further reading

Burke JP, Scott WE, Kutshke PJ. Anterior transposition of the inferior oblique muscle for dissociated vertical deviation. *Ophthalmology* 1993; **100**: 245

Cooper EL, Sandell GS. Recession versus free myotomy at the insertion of the inferior oblique muscle: comparative analysis of the surgical correction of overaction of the inferior oblique muscle. *J Pediatr Ophthalmol* 1969; **6**: 6

Dunlap EA. Inferior oblique weakening. Recession, myotomy, myectomy or disinsertion? *Ann Ophthalmol* 1972; **4**: 905–12

Dyer JA. Tenotomy of the inferior oblique muscle at its scleral insertion. *Arch Ophthalmol* 1962; **68**: 176–81

Fells P. Management of paralytic strabismus. *Br J Ophthalmol* 1974; **58**: 255

Fells P. Surgical management of cyclotorsion. *Int Opthhalmol Clin* 1976; **16**: 161

Harada M, Ito Y. Surgical correction of cyclotropia. *Jap J Ophthalmol* 1964; **8**: 88–96

Harcourt B, Almond S, Freedman H. The efficacy of inferior oblique myectomy operations. In: Mein J, Moore S (eds). *Orthoptics, research and practice. Transactions of the Fourth International Orthoptic Congress, Berne.* Kimpton, London. 1981; 20–3

Helveston EM, Ellis FD. Superior oblique tuck for superior oblique palsy. *Aust J Ophthalmol* 1983; **11**: 215–20

Kushner BJ. Restriction of elevation in abduction after inferior oblique anteriorization. *J Am Assoc Pediatr Ophthalmol Strabismus* 1997; **1**: 55–62

Morris RJ, Scott WE, Keech RV. Superior oblique tuck surgery in the management of superior oblique palsies. *J Pediatr Ophthalmol Strabismus* 1992; **29**: 337

Matthews TD, Patel BCK, Lee JP, Fells P. Disinsertion and recession of the inferior oblique muscle. *Proceedings of the 6th Meeting of the International Strabismological Association, Brussels.* 1992

Mulvihill A, Murphy P, Lee JP. Disinsertion of the inferior oblique muscle for the treatment of superior oblique paresis. *J Pediatr Ophthalmol Strabismus* 2000; **37**: 279–82

14

Adjustable suture techniques

This chapter examines:

Indications for adjustable sutures

The surgical procedure for adjustable sutures

Methods of adjustment

Adjustable suture surgery has become increasingly popular as a way of reducing immediate over- and undercorrections, and therefore helping to provide better long-term stability after squint surgery. Most adults and some older children are suitable for this type of surgery. Adjustable surgery on the rectus muscles (recessions, resections, advancements and transpositions) is straightforward. Adjustable oblique muscle surgery has been described but is rarely attempted.

Adjustable suture surgery

Principles: Surgery is carried out so that, with patient participation, the operated muscles can be moved into the optimum position to ensure the best result with regard to eye position, range of extraocular movements and field of BSV.

Indications: Many surgeons use adjustable sutures as routine for all adult squints in order to reduce the number of re-operations. Consideration of the use of adjustable sutures should take place in the following situations:

- Restrictive strabismus
- Nerve palsies
- Complex strabismus of any description
- Re-operations in adults
- High risk of postoperative diplopia if under- or overcorrected.

Procedure

The amount of surgery performed should be aimed at correcting the squint without adjustment and the adjustable sutures are used as a safety net.

One-step surgery

The entire procedure can be carried out using only topical anaesthesia. This is reasonable for a single rectus muscle recession.

Two-step surgery

Surgery is performed under general anaesthesia, but the extraocular muscles are sutured in such a way as to permit adjustment of the final eye position under topical anaesthesia once the patient has woken up. It is preferable for the patient to have no premedication and a short-acting anaesthetic should be used so that the patient has made a full recovery and is wide awake for the adjustment.

Method

1. Drape the eye and instill adrenaline 0.01% or phenylephrine 2.5% drops to constrict the conjunctival vessels and so reduce bleeding. Place two traction sutures at the 12 and 6 o'clock positions at the limbus.
2. Use two relieving conjunctival incisions, placed slightly more parallel to the muscle borders than in a standard approach, to expose the muscle (Figure 14.1a). If there is extensive conjunctival scarring from previous surgery, open the conjunctiva as close to the limbus as possible.
3. Dissect down the subconjunctival space on either side of the muscle using Westcott scissors in a spreading (not cutting) fashion. Do not dissect directly over the muscle as this tends to bleed.
4. Pass a squint hook into this area and hook the muscle.
5. Clean the Tenon's capsule from the muscle, using blunt dissection, if possible, although in re-do operations scarring may make this impossible and sharp dissection is required.
6. Replace the hook with a Chavasse hook, which spreads the muscle.

Recession/advancement

7. Place two bites of a double-ended 6/0 absorbable suture (dyed polyglycolic acid is the optimum suture as it slides well in the tissues) through the centre third of the insertion of the muscle and tie this (Figure 14.1b). Take a double bite of each outer third of the muscle, one partial thickness and one full thickness, and lock off this suture (Figure 14.1c).

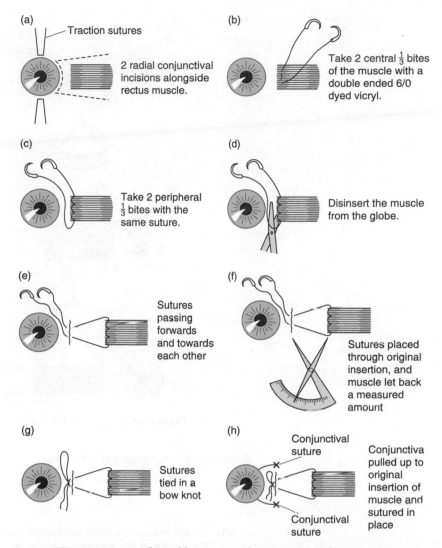

(a) Traction sutures — 2 radial conjunctival incisions alongside rectus muscle.

(b) Take 2 central $\frac{1}{3}$ bites of the muscle with a double ended 6/0 dyed vicryl.

(c) Take 2 peripheral $\frac{1}{3}$ bites with the same suture.

(d) Disinsert the muscle from the globe.

(e) Sutures passing forwards and towards each other

(f) Sutures placed through original insertion, and muscle let back a measured amount

(g) Sutures tied in a bow knot

(h) Conjunctival suture — Conjunctival suture — Conjunctiva pulled up to original insertion of muscle and sutured in place

Figure 14.1 Adjustable suture techniques – muscle recession

8. Detach the muscle from the globe (Figure 14.1d) (go down list to point 11 under 'Recession/advancement and resection').

Resection

9. Place the double-ended 6/0 suture through the belly of the muscle the required number of millimetres to be resected behind the point of insertion, in exactly the same way as for a recession/advancement (above) (Figure 14.2a) (resect 1 mm more than required in order to allow the muscle end to be left a little recessed).

10. Detach the muscle from the globe resecting the appropriate amount of tissue (Figure 14.2b).

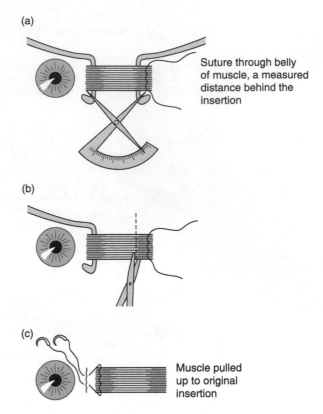

(a)

Suture through belly of muscle, a measured distance behind the insertion

(b)

(c)

Muscle pulled up to original insertion

Figure 14.2   Adjustable suture techniques – resection

Recession/advancement and resection

11. In both resections and recessions pass the two suture ends through the centre of the normal anatomical muscle insertion, about 2 mm apart, placing the sutures so that they are closer together at the anterior aspect than the posterior aspect (Figure 14.1e). For a recession or an advancement the muscle is now positioned the required number of millimetres behind the insertion (Figure 14.1f). For a resection the muscle is pulled up almost to the insertion, as this means that the muscle can either be let back or pulled up to the insertion (Figure 14.2c).

12. Cut the sutures leaving about 4–5 cm spare. Tie the sutures with a bow knot that will be easy to untie (Figure 14.1g).

13. Close the conjunctiva so that the front edge lies just in front of the knotted 6/0 suture (Figure 14.1h) and tuck the loose ends of the suture underneath the conjunctiva, or place in the inferior fornix, or tape to the cheek or forehead with steristrips.

Adjustment procedure (Table 14.1)

- Adjustment can be performed as soon as the patient has recovered from general anaesthesia, but can be delayed for anything up to 2 days postoperatively. If the adjustment is to be carried out soon after the surgery, it is not advisable to use any form of premedication.
- The patient should have the eyes open and moving about for about 30 minutes before the adjustment is carried out (generous amounts of topical anaesthetic make this possible).
- The postoperative position of the eyes, for near and distance, ocular movements and the presence or absence of diplopia in different directions of gaze are assessed prior to the adjustment.
- The patient should wear their normal spectacle correction (Figure 14.3a). Ensure that prisms (if worn) are removed from the lenses.
- The cover test is performed and the patient's ocular movements should be observed in all directions of gaze, since there may be a trade-off between the effect of surgery on the position of the eye, area and location of any field of binocular single vision and any restrictions of movement due to the underlying pathology.

No adjustment required

If no adjustment is necessary and the muscle suture is buried beneath the conjunctiva, no adjustment is required and the patient may be discharged home. Otherwise open the eye with a speculum, cut the loop of

Table 14.1 Key to successful adjustment

---

1 The deviation must be assessed for both near and distance – if the deviation is greater for near rather than distance, carry out the adjustment on the medial rectus and *vice versa*

2 If the field of BSV is limited, try to position it centrally horizontally. Vertically – sacrifice the upper field in order to maximize the field below the midline

3 The eye movements should not be restricted, although in secondary and consecutive exotropias it is beneficial to restrict abduction of the deviating eye slightly at the time of adjustment as this helps to prevent further redivergence

4 Overcorrect consecutive or secondary exotropias if there is no diplopia (although this needs to be cosmetically acceptable). This reduces the risks of later redivergence

5 Leave vertical deviations undercorrected, particularly dysthyroid eye disease and IV nerve palsies

6 In cases with tenuous binocular vision, leave the patient to look around for several minutes to allow them to settle into their new ocular position. Diplopia often settles after a few moments

7 It may be necessary to make adjustments in stages, allowing the patient a short period of stabilization to settle into their new ocular position

8 In cosmetic cases, do not adjust the position based solely on the cover test results, but ensure that the cosmetic appearance is satisfactory. Allow the patient to look in the mirror before tying off the sutures permanently

---

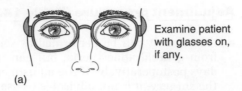

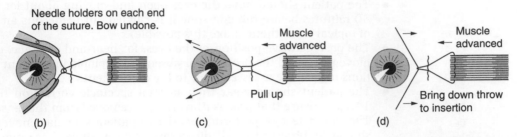

Figure 14.3 Adjustable suture techniques – advancing a recesse muscle

the bow, pull out the loose end and complete the knot. The conjunctiva can be left recessed over the muscle insertion, or may be advanced to the limbus and sutured in place with buried 8/0 absorbable sutures.

Adjustment required

If adjustment is required the following steps are taken:

1. Instill topical anaesthetic (benoxinate, proxymetacaine) several times to ensure good effect
2. Perform the adjustment procedure (see below)
3. Re-test the eye movements and the cover test
4. Instill more anaesthetic and re-adjust if required
5. Repeat as often as required
6. Tie off the sutures and bury the ends
7. Close the conjunctiva if desired
8. Instill topical antibiotic agent.

To advance a muscle

1. Open the eye with a speculum
2. Undo the bow, but leave the first throw of the knot in place
3. Hold each end of the suture with a pair of needle holders close to the eye and pull up these sutures in stages, snugging the knot down to the insertion at each stage (Figure 14.4b–d)
4. Re-bow the knot.

To release a muscle

1. Undo the bow, but leave the first throw of the knot in place.
2. Hold up both ends of the suture with one pair of needle holders and place the closed tips of another needle holder between the globe and

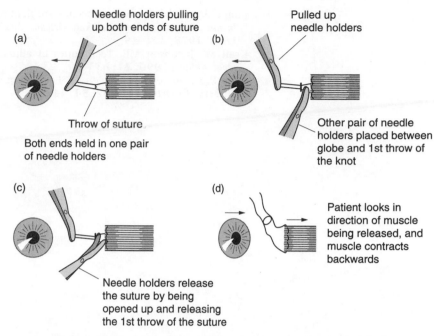

(a)

Needle holders pulling
up both ends of suture

Throw of suture

Both ends held in one pair
of needle holders

(b)

Pulled up
needle holders

Other pair of needle
holders placed between
globe and 1st throw of
the knot

(c)

Needle holders release
the suture by being
opened up and releasing
the 1st throw of the suture

(d)

Patient looks in
direction of muscle
being released, and
muscle contracts
backwards

Figure 14.4 Adjustable suture techniques – releasing a muscle

the first throw of the knot (Figure 14.5a). Open up the needle holder tips to release the suture in small increments (Figure 14.5 b–c).

3. Ask the patient to look in the direction of action of the muscle so that the loose suture is taken up (Figure 14.5d). (If the suture is not taken up by the patient looking in the direction of action of the muscle, it is also possible to release the muscle by pulling some of the suture posteriorly through the insertion.)

4. Re-bow the knot.

Counter traction can be applied by inserting a 'handle suture' at the time of surgery. This is a non-absorbable 6/0 nylon suture that is placed through the insertion of the muscle beside the adjustable suture. This can be used routinely or for those starting to perform adjustable surgery. It is particularly useful when operating upon the superior rectus, as Bell's phenomenon may make access to the muscle difficult.

Further reading

Fells P. Adjustable sutures. *Eye* 1988; **2**: 33–5

Good WV, Hoyt CS. (eds). *Strabismus management*. Butterworth-Heinemann, Boston. 1996

Jampolsky A. Current techniques of adjustable strabismus surgery. *Am J Ophthalmol* 1979; **88**: 406

Jampolsky A. Adjustable strabismus surgical procedures. In *Symposium on strabismus. Transactions of the New Orleans Academy of Ophthalmology*. Mosby, St Louis. 1978; 321–49

Kraft SP, Jacobson ME. Techniques of adjustable suture strabismus surgery. *Ophthal Surg* 1990; **21**: 633

Tiffin PAC, Coyle G, MacEwen CJ. Long-term stability of adjustable strabismus surgery. *Br Orthopt J* 1997; **54**: 44

15

The use of botulinum toxin in the management of strabismus

This chapter examines the uses of botulinum toxin:

Diagnostic purposes

Therapeutic purposes

The methods of extraocular muscle and retrobulbar injection are described

Botulinum toxin is an extremely useful tool in the management of strabismus. The indication for using toxin should be clear prior to giving the injection and further management arranged around the outcome.

Injection of botulinum toxin into an extraocular muscle

Principle

A single extraocular muscle is injected with botulinum toxin which causes weakness of that muscle and an alteration in the alignment of the eyes. The duration of action of the toxin is usually a number of weeks and, after this, the muscle will gradually return to its full strength.

Indications

Diagnostic uses

Botulinum toxin is used diagnostically to assess the binocular sensory and/or motor status, and to evaluate eye movements.

- To assess if troublesome diplopia will occur if squint surgery is performed
  - in cases where the orthoptic postoperative diplopia test is positive
  - in those with constant double vision, which is non-troublesome, but who have a cosmetically poor strabismus. An injection of

toxin will identify if altering the position of the diplopic images will be symptomatic.

- To assess if a patient has useful binocular function (conventional orthoptic testing may fail to detect this).
- To assess the function of a palsied or previously recessed muscle by weakening its ipsilateral antagonist. This is particularly useful in patients with VI nerve palsies, to assess the degree of recovery, or in those who had strabismus surgery in the past and it is not clear whether a reduced movement is due to an overweakened muscle or contracture of the contralateral synergist.
- To identify if a patient with a reduced field of vision has sufficient field to support binocular single vision – especially after a head injury, neurosurgery, retinal surgery or advanced glaucoma.

Therapeutic uses

Botulinum toxin is used to treat a squint.

- Recurrent injections of botulinum toxin improve the ocular deviation in patients for whom no further surgery is deemed possible, usually because of excessive scarring. These injections are usually repeated every 4–6 months.
- In association with rectus muscle transposition surgery in order to weaken an ipsilateral antagonist without interfering with its blood supply (e.g. in unrecovered VI nerve palsies – inject toxin to the medial rectus and transpose the inferior and superior recti laterally).
- Treatment of small postoperative overcorrections in which a functional result was expected (especially after surgery for intermittent exotropia which resulted in an esotropia, with diplopia).
- To effect a functional cure of the strabismus in patients with binocular function, but have a motor cause for their strabismus:
  - to the contracted ipsilateral medial rectus muscle in long-standing, but recovered VI nerve palsy
  - in early cases of thyroid eye disease, with recent onset of strabismus
  - decompensating exo- or esophoria
  - sudden-onset esotropia in children.

In such cases it is not always possible to effect a 'cure', however, in a substantial proportion of such cases control of the deviation is recovered, which may negate the need for surgery.

- To reduce symptoms of an overacting ipsilateral antagonist while awaiting spontaneous recovery from a nerve palsy. This works well in selected individuals with a VI nerve palsy, by injecting the medial rectus, but should only be employed when the underlying cause of the nerve palsy is known, as the toxin may mask the development of fresh neurological signs.
- To reduce symptomatic oscillopsia in cases of acquired nystagmus – a retrobulbar/intraconal injection is used to paralyse all the eye movements. This can only be used for one eye at a time and the

other eye must be covered, as it continues to move, causing intolerable binocular symptoms. Retrobulbar toxin induces a complete ptosis, which should be treated with a ptosis prop. This should be considered as a last resort to reduce symptoms and is not always successful.

Method of injection

Injection of an extraocular muscle

Botulinum toxin is administered on an outpatient basis, under topical anaesthetic.

Children usually require ketamine anaesthesia, but they also need topical anaesthetic as ketamine does not prevent the sensation of pain as the needle enters the subconjunctival space.

All injections should be carried out under electromyographic control, using an EMG machine designed for this purpose. Insulated needles are also used to give the appropriate responses.

Dilution of the botulinum toxin: this is approximately 1/10 the dilution of the recommended dose for orbicularis injection (for blepharospasm). The injected volume is usually 0.1 ml and should be drawn up in a 1 ml syringe for accuracy. There are two types of toxin on the market Botox and Dysport (see below for dilutions).

1. Instill topical anaesthetic (e.g. l benoxinate or proxymetacaine) until the patient feels no more stinging from the drops.
2. Lie the patient on a couch or reclining chair.
3. Place electrodes on the skin, connected to an audio-amplifier/oscilloscope to monitor the EMG signal.
4. Test the electrodes on the skin by getting the patient to wrinkle the forehead in order to stimulate reading from the amplifier.
5. One drop of phenylephrine 2.5% is instilled shortly before giving the injection in order to induce vasoconstriction which reduces the risks of subconjunctival haemorrhage.
6. a) *Medial rectus:*
   - The patient is asked to abduct the eye
   - The needle is inserted subconjunctivally over the approximate area of the insertion of the medial rectus (Figure 15.1a)
   - The patient is asked to adduct the eye
   - Direct the needle posteriorly, in a direction parallel to the medial wall of the orbit towards the apex of the orbit (Figure 15.1b)
   - A loud EMG signal should be heard when the needle is in the region of the motor end plate (Figure 15.1b)
   - It may be necessary to ask the patient to look from side to side on a number of occasions in order to detect maximum firing of the muscle
   - Inject 0.1 ml at this point
   b) *Lateral rectus:*
   - The patient is asked to adduct the eye

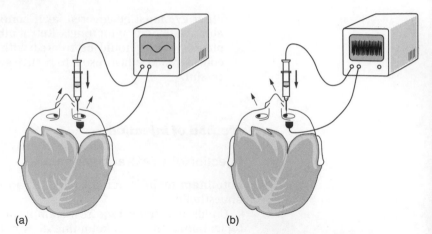

Figure 15.1 Injection of botulinum toxin into the medial rectus

- Insert the needle through the conjunctiva over the insertion of the lateral rectus muscle (Figure 15.2a)
- The patient is asked to abduct the eye and the position of the needle should be moved with the eye
- Direct the needle posteriorly, in a direction parallel to the lateral wall towards the orbital apex, i.e. at about 45° from the midline (Figure 15.2b)
- A loud signal should be heard when the needle is in the correct place
- Inject at this point

c) *Inferior rectus:*
- This can be approached through the inferior fornix, very similar to the approach used for the medial and lateral recti, but more usually the approach is through the lower lid crease directly below the centre of the globe (Figure 15.3a)

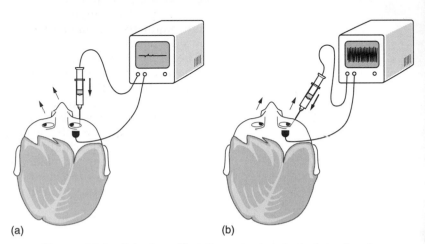

Figure 15.2 Injection of botulinum toxin into the lateral rectus

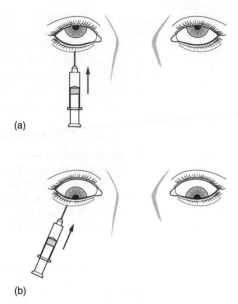

Figure 15.3   Injection of botulinum toxin into the inferior rectus

- The needle is then passed posteriorly and slightly medially towards the orbital apex, along the anatomical line of the muscle (Figure 15.3a)
- The patient is asked to look up and then to look down. A signal heard on upgaze indicates that the needle is close to the inferior oblique – to reach the inferior rectus the needle needs to be inserted further into the orbit until firing is heard on downgaze (Figure 15.3b)
- Inject at this point

d) *The superior rectus* is not a candidate for toxin injection as this induces a ptosis which negates the beneficial effects of the injection

e) *The inferior oblique* may be injected, but the effect is often short lived

f) *The superior oblique* is not a candidate for toxin injection as this induces a ptosis which negates the beneficial effects of the injection.

7. When the tip of the needle is in the correct place, as determined by the EMG, inject 0.1 ml of the diluted botulinum toxin.

8. Keep the needle *in situ* for 45 seconds to 1 minute, so that the drug does not leak along the needle track and affect the other extraocular muscles.

9. Remove the needle.

POSSIBLE COMPLICATIONS OF BOTULINUM TOXIN TREATMENT

- Subconjunctival haemorrhage
- Headache (which settles with simple analgesia)

- Ptosis (which is transient)
- Unwanted deviation (e.g. vertical, when treating a horizontal deviation) due to spread of the toxin to another muscle
- Incomitance (which is less of a problem than might be expected)
- Double vision, which may be troublesome, but is transient
- Perforation of the globe (rare and usually only in high risk cases, e.g. high myopes, or those with excessive scarring)

RETROBULBAR/INTRACONAL INJECTIONS OF BOTULINUM TOXIN

1. No topical anaesthetic is required.
2. Insert a retrobulbar needle through the skin at the inferolateral aspect of the orbit, pass this backwards into the orbit, slightly medially and upwards.
3. Inject 0.4 ml (10 international units).
4. Remove needle immediately.

Dilution and dosage of botulinum toxin

DYSPORT

1. Take a 10 ml vial of N. saline for injection (non-preserved saline)
2. Remove 1 ml from the vial (do not discard the remainder)
3. Add this 1 ml to the vial of saline to reconstitute the dysport toxin
4. Remove 0.5 ml of this reconstituted toxin
5. Add this to the remaining 9 ml of saline – making this up to 9.5 ml
6. This dilution should be used in:
   - 0.1 ml quantities for a rectus muscle providing a dose of 2.5 units of botulinum toxin per injection
   - 0.4 ml quantities for intraconal injections (10 units)

BOTOX

1. Reconstitute the vial of Botox with 4 ml of non-preserved saline
2. Do not shake the bottle after reconstitution
3. This dilution should be used in:
   - 0.1 ml quantities for a rectus muscle providing a dose of 2.5 units of toxin per injection
   - 0.4 ml quantities for intraconal injections (10 units)

Further reading

Elston JS, Lee JP. Paralytic strabismus: the role of botulinum toxin. *Br J Ophthalmol* 1985; **69**: 891–6

Fitzsimmons R, Lee JP, Elston J. Treatment of sixth nerve palsy in adults with combined botulinum toxin chemodenervation and surgery. *Ophthalmology* 1998; **95**: 1535–42

Ketley MJ, Powell CM, Lee JP, Elston J. Botulinum toxin adaptation test: the use of botulinum toxin in the investigation of the sensory state in strabismus. In: Lenk-Schafer M, Calcutt C, Doyle M, Moore S (eds). *Orthoptic horizons. Transac-*

tions of the Sixth International Orthoptic Congress, British Orthoptic Society, London. 1987; 289

Hakin K, Lee JP. Binocular diplopia in unilateral aphakia: the role of botulinum toxin. *Eye* 1991; **5**: 447–50

Heyworth PL, Lee JP. Persisting hypotropias following protective ptosis induced by botulinum neurotoxin. *Eye* 1994; **8**: 551–5

Horgan SE, Lee JP, Bunce C. The longterm use of botulinum toxin for adult straismus. *J Pediatr Ophthalmol Strabismus* 1998; **35**: 9–16

Lee JP, Elson J, Vickers S et al. Botulinum toxin therapy for squint. *Eye* 1988; **2**: 24–8

Lee JP. Modern management of sixth nerve palsy. *Aust NZ J Ophthalmol* 1992; **20**: 41–46

Lymburn EG, MacEwen CJ. Botulinum toxin in the management of heterophoria. *Br Orthoptic J* 1994; **51**: 38

Lymburn EG, MacEwen CJ. Diagnostic applications of botulinum toxin: regarding the sensory status of patients with strabismus. *Br Orthoptic J* 1998; **55**: 45–7

Lyons CJ, Vickers S, Lee JP. Botulinum toxin in dysthyroid strabismus. *Eye* 1990; **4**: 538–42

Rayner SA, Hollick EJ, Lee JP. Botulinum toxin in childhood strabismus. *Strabismus* 1999; **7**: 103–11

Ruben ST, Lee JP, O'Neil D, Dunlop I, Elston JS. The use of botulinum toxin for treatment of acquired nystagmus and oscillopsia. *Ophthalmology* 1994; **101**: 783–7

Scott AB, Magoon EH, McNeer KW, Stager DR. Botulinum toxin treatment of childhood strabismus. *Ophthalmology* 1990; **27**: 1434–8

Scott AB. Botulinum toxin injection into extra ocular muscles as an alternative to strabismus surgery. *Ophthalmology* 1980; **87**: 1044–9

Scott AB, Rosenbaum AL, Collins CC. Pharmacological weakening of the extra-ocular muscles. *Invest Ophthalmol Vis Sci* 1973; **2**: 924–9

16

Complications of strabismus surgery – how to avoid and manage them

> Complications are classified as:
>
> **Peroperative**
>
> **Immediate postoperative**
>
> **Late postoperative**
>
> This chapter covers the identification and management of slipped and detached extraocular muscles

Serious complications associated with strabismus surgery are fortunately uncommon. Less severe problems may occur with more frequency either during or after surgery. Patients should be advised of the risks of these complications, which may differ, depending on each particular operation.

Peroperative complications

Surgery to the wrong muscle

This may be due either to a pre- or peroperative problem.

Preoperative cause

Occasionally surgery is performed on the wrong muscle due to administrative error, with incorrect identification of the patient or failure to check which eye is to undergo surgery.

AVOIDANCE

This is best avoided by a clear instruction in the notes as to which muscles require surgery and by what amounts, written in longhand, when the patient is assessed.

MANAGEMENT

As soon as the error is recognized corrective surgery should be carried out, by reversing the surgery if possible.

Peroperative cause

The wrong muscle may be picked up and operated on if the surgical exposure is inadequate. This is most likely to be confusion between the inferior oblique and the adjacent lateral or inferior rectus muscles.

AVOIDANCE

- If there is any doubt about the identity of a muscle that has been hooked through a conjunctival wound, the surgeon can give the muscle a gentle tug and see the effect upon the eye. If, for example, the inferior rectus has been hooked instead of the inferior oblique, pulling the hook will not elevate the eye. Alternatively, the adjacent muscles should be clearly identified by increasing the size of the conjunctival incision to confirm that the correct muscle is undergoing surgery.
- Some patients, commonly those with craniofacial dysostoses, can have whole orbits that are excyclotorted. This can mean that the rectus muscles insert into the globe in unexpected locations and can lead to confusion between them. Preoperative knowledge of this potential problem and consideration of it is usually enough to allow the surgeon to identify the muscles correctly.

MANAGEMENT

As soon as the error is recognized corrective surgery should be carried out, by reversing the surgery if possible.

Globe perforation

Cause

1. During the detachment of a tight or scarred muscle from the globe.
2. During suturing of the muscle to the globe.

AVOIDANCE

1. Take care during muscle detachment, especially in cases of restrictive strabismus and in re-operations. Do not 'tent up' the sclera attachment of the muscle when cutting the muscle from its insertion.
2. If access for a recession is poor, or if the surgeon is especially inexperienced, perform a hang back recession.

MANAGEMENT

- Continue with the strabismus surgery.
- Give subconjunctival antibiotics at the end of surgery.

- Examine fundus via dilated pupil either in operating theatre or post-operatively.
- Retinal cryotherapy is unnecessary.

In the rare event that there is a macroscopic defect in the sclera, this should be repaired using the operating microcscope, having removed any prolapsed vitreous.

Haemorrhage

CAUSES

1. Significant haemorrhage rarely complicates squint surgery, although excessive oozing may promote scar tissue and care should be taken to reduce bleeding from all sites.
2. Excessive bleeding can sometimes be a problem in re-operations with vascularized and scarred conjunctiva.
3. Inferior oblique surgery where muscle, rather than tendon, is cut, is prone to haemorrhage, unless appropriate steps are taken to prevent this.
4. Rupture of a vortex vein may occur when operating on the superior rectus or superior oblique.

AVOIDANCE

1. The use of gentle diathermy is essential to keep the operative field free of blood. Diathermy to obvious vessels prior to cutting or placing sutures is recommended.
2. The use of vasoconstrictors such as adrenaline or phenylephrine drops applied immediately prior to surgery and careful diathermy during the surgery reduce this problem of increased bleeding.
3. The inferior oblique muscle should be firmly held until it is clear that all bleeding points have been secured. If the muscle is allowed to retract into the orbit immediately after detachment from the sclera, it may be difficult to locate and a significant haematoma may occur.
4. Care must be taken, when exposing these muscles, to identify the vortex veins and carefully to preserve them.

MANAGEMENT

If a significant haemorrhage occurs it is best to identify the cause and attempt to stop bleeding from the source. If a significant haematoma develops, an expectant policy is adopted and it usually settles within 10–14 days. Bleeding from the inferior oblique may predispose to an adherence syndrome (see below).

Detached muscle

A muscle that is 'detached' or 'lost' has become free from the globe, with no attachments remaining. This usually becomes evident at the time of surgery, when the muscle that is undergoing surgery slips from the sutures that were holding it, or is cut free from the eye. Occasionally this presents as an early postoperative complication, when the muscle appears to be sutured to the globe at the end of surgery, but on postoperative examination there is no function of the affected muscle, and exploration indicates that it is no longer attached to the globe.

CAUSES

A muscle may slip off the sutures that are holding it after it has been disinserted from the globe. More rarely, a muscle may spontaneously rupture or tear during surgery. The muscle then retracts backwards into its sleeve of Tenon's capsule.

AVOIDANCE

● Careful suture placement.
● Ensure that the entire muscle is included in the suture.
● Do not place the suture too near the end of the muscle.
● Do not cut the muscle too close to the attached sutures.
● Ensure good firm bites when suturing the muscle to the sclera.
● Do not tug or jerk muscles during surgery.

MANAGEMENT

This complication requires urgent and immediate attention as the optimum time to relocate the muscle is at the time of surgery. The lost muscle retracts into the orbit down its sheath in Tenon's capsule (Figure 16.1a).

● DO NOT – pull on Tenon's capsule (Figure 16.1b).
● DO NOT – immediately rotate the eye away from the involved muscle (Figure 16.1d). This is reflex in order to improve exposure, but should be avoided.
● DO – compress the eye against the opposite orbital wall, retroplace the globe and gently open up the Tenon's capsule (Figure 16.1c).
● The plane of dissection should follow this line towards the apex of the orbit (Figure 16.1e) and NOT follow the line of the globe (Figure 16.1f).
● Malleable retractors are helpful in exposing the operation site.
● A headlight will help to improve illumination of the site.
● Recruitment of an extra assistant is very useful, as an extra pair of hands can hold on to the retractors.
● If there is some doubt whether it is muscle or connective tissue that has been discovered, pulling the tissue may induce a bradycardia which assists in the identification of muscle tissue (if the patient has not been atropinized).

The superior and lateral rectus muscles tend not to retract into the orbit because of their attachments to the oblique muscles. The inferior rectus may have some attachment to the inferior oblique and is therefore slightly easier to find than the medial rectus, which has no attachments at all.

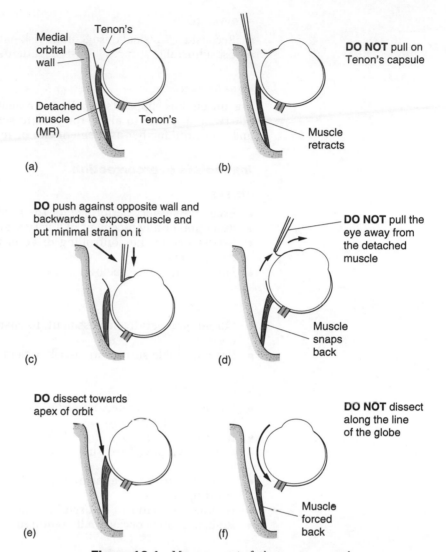

Figure 16.1 Management of a lost rectus muscle

Early postoperative complications

Immediate undercorrection

CAUSES

- Insufficient surgery performed for the angle of the squint.
- Scarred muscle inadequately recessed to permit ocular rotation.
- Excessive drive to squint (e.g. in nystagmus blockage, high AC/A ratio).
- Slipped muscle (see below and Figure 16.2).

AVOIDANCE

- Reconsider surgical dosage in at-risk patients.
- Use adjustable sutures in at-risk patients.

MANAGEMENT

If a muscle has slipped (see below), immediate re-operation is required, otherwise it is best to allow the eyes to settle down after their surgery and wait until further assessment can be made.

Immediate overcorrection

CAUSES

- Excessive surgery performed for the angle of the squint.
- Resection or advancement of a very scarred, tight, muscle.
- Persistence of the controlling drive of pre-existing phoria/intermittent tropia.
- Slipped muscle (see below).

AVOIDANCE

- Careful preoperative assessment, to ensure most appropriate surgical doses.
- Use adjustable sutures in at-risk patients.

MANAGEMENT

- If a muscle has slipped, immediate re-operation is required (see below and Figure 16.2).
- If no suggestion of a slipped muscle, it is best to allow the eyes to settle down after their surgery and wait until further assessment can be made.
- Patching, prisms or altering spectacle correction may be useful in the short term.
- Botulinum toxin can be useful in the longer term.
- Re-operation is occasionally required.

The slipped muscle

An operated muscle may slip from the globe in the immediate postoperative period. There are three possible causes:

1. Failure of the sutures to include all the fibres of the muscle and only the capsule of the muscle has been secured. When the patient moves the eye, the muscle fibres contract backwards inside the capsule, losing contact with the globe and become effectively weakened (Figure 16.2 a i).
2. One of the sutures holding the muscle in place becomes disinserted (Figure 16.2b i).
3. Both of the sutures securing the muscle to the globe become disinserted – effectively a 'lost muscle' (see above and Figure 16.1).

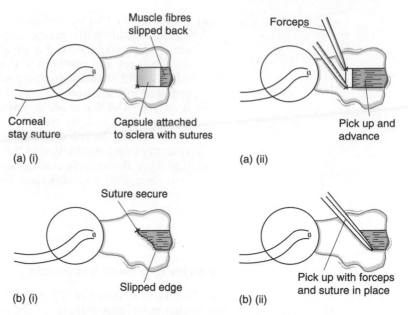

Muscle fibres
slipped back

Forceps

Corneal
stay suture

Capsule attached
to sclera with sutures

Pick up and
advance

(a) (i)

(a) (ii)

Suture secure

Slipped edge

Pick up with forceps
and suture in place

(b) (i)

(b) (ii)

Figure 16.2   Management of a slipped rectus muscle

CLINICAL FEATURES

Immediate postoperative examination reveals weakness of ductions in the direction of gaze. The eye is usually deviated away from the affected muscle.

AVOIDANCE

- Careful placement of sutures, both through the muscle and into the sclera.
- Inspection of the muscle to ensure that it is securely attached to the eye prior to closing the conjunctiva.

MANAGEMENT

Surgical exploration of the muscle should take place immediately – the sooner the muscle is secured the better the prognosis.

1. Place a traction suture through the limbus or cornea in the area of the missing muscle.
2. Cut the conjunctival sutures and open the conjunctival wound. This may be quite adherent, even within 24 hours of initial surgery.
3. Dissect around the muscle very carefully. Great care must be taken not to dislodge any remaining sutures while carrying out the dissection. Do not pass a muscle hook as this may serve to disrupt any remaining sutures.
4. Identify any remaining sutures and any remaining muscle should be attached to these (Figure 16.2a i and ii).

a) If the muscle has slipped inside its capsule (Figure 16.2 a i), pick up the capsule with forceps and advance it until the muscle fibres are evident (Figure 16.2 a ii). Secure the muscle, once identified, with sutures and reattach to the globe in the appropriate position with scleral sutures. If using adjustable sutures these should be replaced in the usual way (see Chapter 14).

b) If only part of the muscle remains attached to the sclera (Figure 16.2 b i) it is usually straightforward to identify the slipped half. This should be picked up with forceps (Figure 16.2 b ii), resutured and reattached to the sclera.

c) If neither the muscle nor the capsule can be found then exploration should be undertaken as for the 'lost muscle' (see above and Figure 16.1).

Anterior segment ischaemia

Significant loss of anterior segment blood supply occurs when more than two rectus muscles are detached from the eye during surgery. High-risk procedures include transposition procedures, surgery on patients with abnormal anatomy and vertical rectus muscle surgery on patients who have previously undergone horizontal surgery. There is hypertrophy of the remaining long posterior ciliary arteries so that after three months more rectus muscle surgery can be performed.

CLINICAL FEATURES

- Ocular pain – which may be severe and persistent.
- Blurred vision.
- Corneal thickening, haze and Descemet's membrane folds.
- Anterior chamber flare.
- Soft eye with a deep anterior chamber.

AVOIDANCE

- Stage surgery.
- Use botulinum toxin to weaken muscles when more than 2 muscles require surgery.

MANAGEMENT

- Intensive topical steroids.
- Analgesics.
- Anterior segment ischaemia is rarely very serious and usually recovers after a few weeks. A short course of systemic steroids may be required.

Prolapsed Tenon's capsule

CLINICAL FEATURES

Tenon's capsule remains exposed and results in a white unsightly scar in the region of the conjunctival incision.

AVOIDANCE

This is caused by failure to oppose conjunctiva to conjunctiva at the end of surgery and it can be avoided by carefully identifying these tissues and closing them carefully.

MANAGEMENT

If a lump of Tenon's capsule is exposed this should be excised under general (children) or local anaesthetic.

Inclusion of plica semilunaris in conjunctival closure

When the medial rectus has been resected, the overlying conjunctiva sometimes appears excessive. The plica semilunaris may be mistaken for the conjunctival edge and sutured to the conjunctiva at the limbus. This causes a cosmetically unsightly scar which may restrict eye movements.

AVOIDANCE

Careful identification of the edge of the conjunctiva and plica when closing conjunctiva after medial rectus surgery (particularly resection or advancement as the conjunctiva may become bunched up in these procedures).

MANAGEMENT

The conjunctiva should be opened and the correct conjunctival edge attached at the limbus. This may not be possible, in which case the conjunctival edge should be recessed.

Conjunctival inclusion cyst

If the edges of the conjunctiva are not closed carefully then a small area of conjunctiva may be buried in the wound. This may cause an inclusion cyst, which is a translucent rounded cyst that is non-tender.

AVOIDANCE

Close edges of conjunctiva carefully.

MANAGEMENT

The lesion should be surgically excised.

Diplopia

Some patients may be troubled in the early postoperative period by diplopia. This may have been predicted by preoperative testing and in some cases botulinum toxin may have been administered to determine the effect of this diplopia. In other cases, which may have been unpredicted, an area of unsuppressed retina has been exposed or there has been an inability to suppress.

AVOIDANCE

Use diagnostic botulinum toxin in cases where there is risk of postoperative diplopia.

MANAGEMENT

* This should be left to settle spontaneously, either by suppression (in children and some adults) or by adaptation to the situation.
* Patching may be required in the acute phase.
* In some cases further treatment to alter the deviation is required, although the results of this cannot be guaranteed.
* In cases that have become insuperable and untreatable it may be necessary to occlude the affected eye with a patch, occlusive spectacle, contact or intraocular lens (this is very rare).

Postoperative infection

Various forms of infection are recognized following squint surgery. They usually manifest themselves within the first 5–7 postoperative days. Serious infection is rare.

Conjunctivitis

A mild inflammation is common postoperatively but occasionally this becomes secondarily infected causing a mild conjunctivitis.

AVOIDANCE

Use preoperative conjunctival povidone iodine and postoperative topical antibiotics.

MANAGEMENT

This responds well to topical antibiotics (which some use routinely postoperatively for 1–2 weeks).

Orbital cellulitis

This presents with pain, lid swelling and pyrexia.

AVOIDANCE

Use preoperative conjunctival povidone iodine, postoperative topical antibiotics.

MANAGEMENT

This usually responds well to systemic antibiotics.

Endophthalmitis

This is a very rare complication. The risks are thought to be increased if the sclera is perforated at the time of surgery.

AVOIDANCE

Use preoperative conjunctival povidone iodine, postoperative topical antibiotics.

MANAGEMENT

Intravitreal antibiotics.
    Vitrectomy in cases where the vision falls to the level of perception of light or less.

Suture granuloma

This problem was commoner in the past when catgut sutures were used. A raised, red area appears in the region of the suture a few weeks post-operatively.

AVOIDANCE

- Use modern absorbable (polyglycolic acid) sutures to close conjunctiva (preferably 8.0).
- Bury conjunctival sutures.

MANAGEMENT

This may improve with topical steroids but may require surgical removal.

Dellen

Corneal dellen may develop if there is marked conjunctival swelling at the limbus. This is commoner after re-operations. An area of corneal thinning develops due to poor wetting of the cornea.

AVOIDANCE

- Bury conjunctival sutures carefully. Oppose conjunctival tissues at close of surgery.

MANAGEMENT

- Topical steroids may reduce the swelling.
- Topical lubricants are used until the conjunctival swelling has settled.

Late complications

Inferior oblique adherence syndrome

Violation of Tenon's capsule with fat prolapse into the operative site may lead to the formation of dense scar tissue. This occurs predominantly after surgery to the inferior oblique. The eye is progressively pulled downwards and cannot be elevated on forced duction test.

AVOIDANCE

Always identify the inferior oblique clearly before trying to pick it up and never try to hook it blindly.

MANAGEMENT

This is very difficult to treat effectively but recession of the ipsilateral inferior rectus may improve the situation, combined with division of adhesions and scar tissue.

Late re-operation

CAUSES FOR THE NEED FOR RE-OPERATION

1. Initial surgery was an over- or undercorrection – which may be due to inappropriate surgery or due to an unusual reaction to the surgery.
2. The complexity and the unpredictability of outcome determines that surgery needs to be staged (this will usually have been decided prior to initial surgery).
3. Absence of binocular function causes an unstable alignment.
4. Disease process remits or relapses (e.g. dysthyroid eye disease).
5. Scarring causes changes in the balance of orbital forces.

MANAGEMENT

1. When assessing a patient for re-operation, it is important to establish which of the above underlying factors is present.
2. If an unexpected result has occurred following surgery, it is not possible to correct it by simply undoing the previous surgery. Any

decision about further surgery should be based on the 'current' findings, together with knowledge of previous operations performed (if this is known and some educated guesses may be required).

3. In some instances the final decision regarding surgical approach may only be made after the muscles have been surgically explored and their exact location identified.

4. It may be necessary to operate on both eyes, in order to correct the alignment without producing severe restriction of movements. It is essential that patients are made aware of this possibility prior to surgery and are consented appropriately.

SURGERY

1. Conjunctival incision – this may be difficult because of conjunctival adherence from previous surgery.

2. Perform forced duction tests to confirm or exclude muscle tightness.

3. Dissect down on either side of the muscle breaking down adhesions and dealing with bleeding points.

4. Hook muscle – if muscle has been previously recessed then this may hook a 'false' tendon where the conjunctiva is adherent to the original insertion.

5. Gently dissect down on to the hooked tissue using blunt dissection techniques. There may be masses of scar tissue and dissection around each side of the muscle is essential.

6. Clean up the surface of the muscle – some sharp dissection with scissors may be required at this point.

7. Place muscles on adjustable sutures, if possible, as the results of surgery on scarred and contracted muscles are always unpredictable.

Further reading

Apple DJ, Jones GR, Reidy JJ, Loftfield K. Ocular perforation and phthisis bulbi secondary to strabismus surgery. *J Pediatr Ophthalmol Strabismus* 1985; **22**: 184–7

Apt L, Isenberg SJ. The oculocardic reflex as a surgical aid in identifying a slipped or 'lost' extraocular muscle. *Br J Ophthalmol* 1980; **64**: 362–5

Girard LJ, Beltranena F. Early and late complications of extensive muscle surgery. *Arch Ophthalmol* 1960; **64**: 576–84

Good WV, Hoyt CS (eds). *Strabismus Management*. Butterworth-Heinemann. 1995

Gottlieb F, Castro JL. Perforation of the globe during strabismus surgery. *Arch Ophthalmol* 1970; **84**: 151–7

Greenberg DR, Ellenhorn NL, Chapman LI *et al*. Posterior chamber hemorrhage during strabismus surgery. *Am J Ophthalmol* 1988; **106**: 534–5

Helveston EM. Slipped inferior rectus after adjustable sutures. In: Lenk-Schafer M, Calcutt C, Doyle M, Moore S (eds). *Orthoptic horizons. Transactions of the 6th International Orthoptic Congress, Harrogate*. British Orthoptic Society, London. 1987; 421–6

MacEwen CJ, Lee JP, Fells P. Aetiology and management of the 'detached' rectus muscle. *Br J Ophthalmol* 1992; **76**: 131–6

McKeown CA, Lambert HM, Shore JW. Preservation of the anterior ciliary vessels during extra-ocular muscle surgery. *Ophthalmology* 1989; **96**: 498–506

Morris RJ, Rosen PH, Fells P. Incidence of inadvertent globe perforations during strabismus surgery. *Br J Ophthalmol* 1990; **74**: 490–3

Olver JM, Lee JP. Recovery of anterior segment circulation after strabismus surgery in adult patients. *Ophthalmology* 1992; **99**: 305–15

Plager DA, Parks MM. Recognition and repair of the 'lost' rectus muscle. A report of 25 cases. *J Ped Ophthalmol Strabismus* 1990; **97**: 131–7

Plager DA, Parks MM. Recognition and repair of the 'slipped' rectus muscle. *J Ped Ophthalmol Strabismus* 1988; **25**: 270–4

Salamon SM, Friberg TR, Luxenberg MN. Endophthalmitis after strabismus surgery. *Am J Ophthalmol* 1982; **93**: 39

Simon JW, Lininger LL, Scherage JL. Recognized scleral perforation during eye muscle surgery: incidence and sequelae. *J Paediatr Ophthalmol Strabismus* 1992: **29**: 273–5

Appendix – How much muscle surgery is required?

Each patient requires an individual surgical approach to the management of their squint, but the following measurements may be of assistance as a guide, particularly for those beginning strabismus surgery.

For horizontal deviations

- The measurements suggested are only for concomitant deviations, with no underlying muscle or neurological pathology or previous surgery
- The measurements for recessions are taken from the insertion of the muscle
- The measurements should be altered based on audit of the surgeon's personal results
- If the horizontal angle is greater for near than distance relatively more should be done to the medial rectus than the lateral rectus, and vice versa
- For angles >50 dioptres perform bilateral surgery to more than 2 horizontal recti

Eso-deviations

Angle of squint	Bilat. MR recessions	*or*	MR recession/LR resection	
20 D	3.5 mm		4 mm	5 mm
30 D	4.5 mm		5 mm	6 mm
40 D	5 mm		5 mm	7.5 mm
50 D	6 mm		5.5 mm	8 mm

For eso-deviations

- If the AC/A ratio is high (>5 : 1) in a child with an accommodative esotropia, bilateral medial recessions of at least 5 mm should be undertaken, even for small deviations
- Aim to slightly undercorrect secondary esotropia, or those with poor binocular function

Exo-deviations

Angle of squint	Bilat. LR recessions	*or*	LR recession/MR resection	
20 D	5 mm		5 mm	4 mm
30 D	6.5 mm		6.5 mm	5 mm
40 D	8 mm		8 mm	5 mm
50 D	9.5 mm		9 mm	5.5 mm

For exo-deviations

- Exotropias with lateral incomitance require 1mm less recession to the lateral rectus
- Aim to overcorrect consecutive and secondary exotropia.

Vertical deviations

It is much more difficult to provide guidance tables for vertical deviations as they are less likely than horizontal squints to be fully concomitant.

a) In concomitant deviations, the balance between the vertical rectus muscles (which elevate and depress the eye in abduction) and the obliques (which elevate and depress in adduction) must be maintained – always work on ipsilateral antagonists or contralateral synergists

b) As a rule of thumb for vertical recti – recess *1 mm for every 3 dioptres* of height in the primary position – this *increases to 5 dioptres/mm in the field of gaze* (e.g. for deviations in downgaze when operating on the inferior rectus)

c) An *inferior oblique* disinsertion will reduce the size of the vertical angle in the primary position by approximately *12 dioptres*

d) Late overcorrection is a common problem following recessions of the inferior rectus – great care must be taken with this muscle and aim to be conservative

e) Aim to correct a vertical deviation in downgaze principally; upgaze is much less important

f) Always undercorrect long-standing vertical deviations, especially due to thyroid eye disease and 'congenital' IV nerve palsies

Effect of horizontal muscle surgery on A or V patterns

a) *Elevation or depression of contralateral MRs or LRs (move MRs towards the apex of the pattern and vice versa for the LRs)*

- Half width elevation or depression – collapses pattern by 10 dioptres

- Full width elevation or depression – collapses pattern by up to 20 dioptres

b) Graded replacement of the muscles

- A 2 mm difference between the upper and lower borders of both muscles collapses up to 15 dioptres of A or V pattern
- A 3 mm difference between the upper and lower borders of both muscles collapses 20–25 dioptres of A or V pattern

Expect relatively more effect for the surgical amounts for larger pattern deviations.

Index

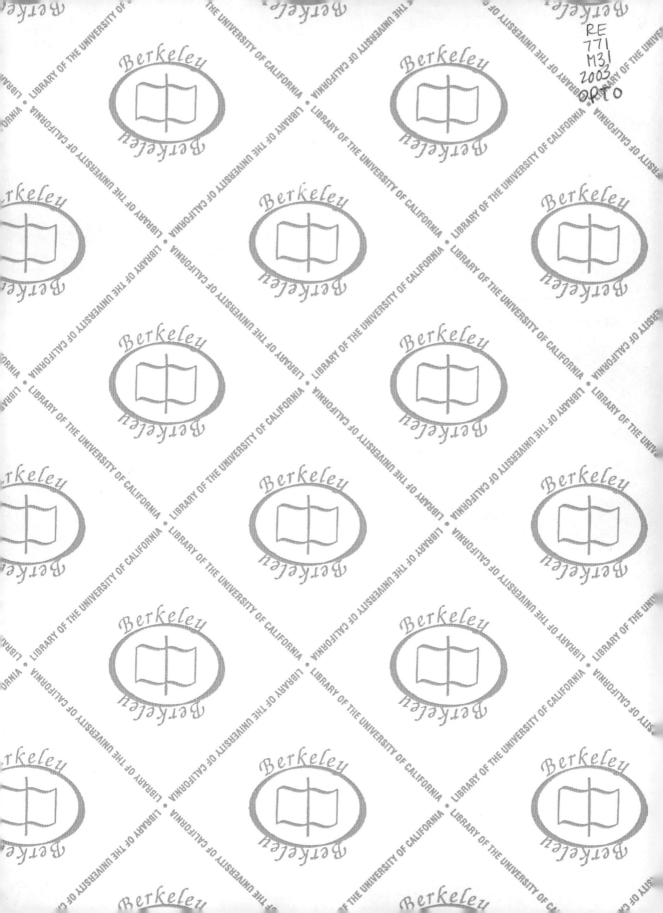